MW01168531

Rutstein

on

Fitness

*Strengthening the Body
to Heal the Mind*

Custom Fitness
Boston, Massachusetts

Rutstein on Fitness: Strengthening the Body to Heal the Mind

©2005 by Jeff Rutstein. All rights reserved. No part of this book may be reproduced or transmitted in any form or by any means, electronic or mechanical, including photo-copying, recording or by any information storage and retrieval system, without written permission from the author, except for the inclusion of brief quotations in a review.

Published by
  Custom Fitness
  75 Saint Alphonsus St., Suite G
  Boston, Massachusetts 02120
  1-800-374-9959
  www.rutsteinonfitness.com

Edited by Patricia Amend
Cover and interior design and layout by Robert Goodman, Silvercat™, San Diego, California

ISBN: 0-9760170-1-6
LCCN: 2004111011

Printed in the United States of America

Jeff Rutstein's book promotes exercise in a measured approach that encourages people to use his methods to promote healing and build psychological and spiritual strength. . . . I strongly recommend to my patients that they read this book in it's entirety and put Mr. Rutstein's lessons to work in their lives.

       ❧ David J. Sugarbaker, M.D.
           Professor of Surgery, Harvard Medical School

. . . a whole new approach to weightlifting . . . exhaling tension on each exertion and inhaling strength on each release.

       ❧ The Washington Post

Rutstein on Fitness is absolutely amazing. Jeff's fitness and lifestyle philosophy will lead many to physical and mental fitness.

       ❧ Wayne L. Westcott, Ph.D.
           author of *Strength Training for Seniors*,
           former advisor to The President's Council
           on Physical Fitness

Rutstein shares his road to recovery with others . . . a kinder, gentler workout.

       ❧ Reuters

With caring, empathy and candor, Jeff genuinely connects with readers who desperately need to feel that someone understands where they are coming from. Having walked in their shoes, Jeff offers readers hope, and more importantly, a practical plan of action that can put them on the path to recovery . . . starting today.

       ❧ Patricia Amend
           co-author of *The 30-Minute Fitness Solution*

The day you realize you are a divine child loved by us and your Creator, Jeff's book will help guide you to a new life.

       ❧ Bernie Siegel, M.D.
           author of *Love, Medicine & Miracles*

Rutstein shares his hard-won wisdom in this clear, easy-to-follow book. His emphasis on "mindful movement" to reduce stress and feel better is a refreshing and welcome change from many exercise books that focus solely on appearance.

                  ✺ Carol Krucoff, co-author of *Healing Moves*
                      founding Health Editor of *The Washington Post*

Jeff has forged his skills as a fitness guru in the crucible of his own struggle to reclaim control of his life. . . . In his straightforward, unpretentious manner, Jeff imparts his knowledge of fitness, nutrition, and health (mental and physical).

                  ✺ Aaron Nelson, Ph.D.
                      Chief of Neuropsychology
                      Brigham and Women's Hospital

In this type of weight training, you have to feel your body work. Your mind and body start to reconnect and it feels great!

                  ✺ *Natural Health*

. . . the fitness industry's best advertisement for the mind/body benefits of regular exercise.

                  ✺ *Club Business International*

If you suffer from depression or related problems, you need to know what is in this book.

                  ✺ Harrison G. Pope, Jr., M.D.
                      Professor of Psychiatry, Harvard Medical School

To call this an exercise book would be akin to calling an F-15 jet fighter a nice little plane.

                  ✺ Alexander Vuckovic, M.D.
                      co-author of *Under Observation*

to the memory

of

my hero and inspiration

my father

Contents

Acknowledgments

It is not possible to mention all the people who have supported and influenced my work. But I must make a special note of Dr. Alec Bodkin who I want to thank for trusting his patients with me and supporting my efforts over the years.

This book project was influenced by many people who have helped me create a vision. They include:

Steve Wagner, who helped me see the larger picture, and has always taken the time to give advice.

Seth Miller, for taking on the role of coach of this book project and leading me in the right direction.

Patricia Amend, who has been the perfect collaborator and editor.

Alec Sohmer, for his expert legal advice.

Antoinette Kuritz, for helping me set a vision and creating a marketing plan to help others achieve joy through exercise.

Bob Goodman, who did such a wonderful job formatting the book.

Kim Tyler, for photographing the interior pictures.

My mother, who made it clear to me that this book had to get done.

Lastly, to my wife, Kerry, who supported my efforts with this book project and continues to give her support and patience.

Foreword

by J. Alexander Bodkin, M.D.

Anxiety and depression are among the most common afflictions facing the human race. Add alcohol and drug abuse, and you are talking about problems that face close to half the population of the United States, at some point in life.

Many remedies have been offered over the years for these often crippling problems. These days, medicines have come to predominate in the treatment of depression and anxiety, as have support groups for addiction problems. A great variety of individual and group psychotherapies are also available and are widely used to help individuals cope with these difficulties.

But one very effective approach has been unaccountably neglected: strength training.

In my clinical work with people suffering from mood and anxiety problems, and the substance abuse that often follows from these, I have found time and time again that consistent, reasonable exercise is a great help. By the time people get to me as patients, exercise alone is no longer enough, but it remains a critical component of a total treatment program. Exercise will hasten recovery, improve well being, increase stress tolerance, relieve physical discomforts, improve physical health and appearance, and boost self-esteem and self-confidence.

The problem is that when people are feeling negatively about themselves, and often painfully self-conscious, going to a gym is the last thing they want to do. For one thing, they wouldn't know where to begin. It just seems like one more opportunity to fail and to be found wanting—in public. The task I face is to get them beyond that point—and my main resource has been to refer them to Jeff Rutstein for consultation and guidance.

Obviously, that is not a resource available to large numbers of people facing these difficult problems, and this book provides a very positive, new alternative.

Some of the ways a well-designed fitness program helps depression and related conditions are:

- ✤ It expresses self-worth—that a person's own body is worth a concerted effort to strengthen and improve.
- ✤ It offers concrete and plain-to-see evidence of progress—the weight you can move with each muscle group steadily advances as long as you just stay at it—as do the distance you can run and the miles you can bike and the laps you can swim.
- ✤ Appearance improves—the physical consequences of passive self-neglect are quite visible. Likewise,

they are also quite visible when self-neglect is replaced by proper self-care.

+ Physical comfort improves—the aches and pains and fatigue that typically accompany anxiety and depression become less and less noticeable.

+ Sleep improves when a person tires himself or herself out with healthy physical exertion.

+ The mind is redirected from troubling thoughts to the task at hand—offering some of the benefits of meditation.

+ After a workout, a person has a much greater capacity to relax—where before they may have felt only tension.

+ Compulsive eating typically drops away with exercise— to be replaced by a healthy appetite for what the body actually needs.

+ Biologically, exercise causes the brain to release neurotransmitters known as endorphins and enkephalins, natural compounds that relieve pain both in the body and in the psyche.

It is true that exercise alone will not suffice if depressive feelings, anxious worries, and the destructive self-treatment of these problems through substance abuse have reached a level of severity that requires professional help. However, if these problems are addressed early enough, then following a healthy, carefully thought-out fitness program may be all that is needed. The use of more invasive treatments—from antidepressants to psychotherapy—may then never become necessary.

This book puts a carefully thought-out, safe, and do-able fitness program at the fingertips of people who need it. The personal odyssey it relates is compelling, and the stories of success from a series of Jeff's clients encourage the reader to give this approach a try. Jeff is doing a public service by making his physical approach to mental health available to a much wider community.

J. Alexander Bodkin, M.D.
Chief, Clinical Psychopharmacology Research Program
McLean Hospital
Belmont, Massachusetts

Introduction

When you hear the term weightlifting, what do you most often think of?

For most people, the phrases *weightlifting, strength training*, and *pumping iron* conjure up images of "meatheads" with bulging muscles strutting along the beach. I was once a meathead.

Unfortunately, this stereotypical image has kept many of us away from a healthy activity that could change our lives. I'm going to ask you to do one important thing right now—that is, forget the pumping iron image forever. Light the fuse, cover your ears, and blow it to pieces. After reading this book you will think about strength training with a whole new mind-set.

I will show you a different approach to strength training that can evolve into a life-altering experience. It isn't just about muscles. When done correctly, it's about rebuilding a foundation of mental and physical strength. It's about regaining health and self-respect. It's about feeling a sense of strength that emanates from your body and permeates your psyche.

The program that I set forth in this book is one that all people, young or old, male or female, can adapt to fit their lives. Studies show that women as well as men gain tremendous health benefits from strength training. Women between 50 and 70 years old will increase their bone density by 1 percent per year if they lift weights regularly, according to a study done by researchers at Tufts University in Boston. Those who don't lift weights lose an average of 2.5 percent bone density per year. This can be a critical difference considering that according to the National Institutes of Health, 10 million individuals, mostly women, have osteoporosis, and 18 million more have low bone mass, placing them at increased risk for this disease. Moreover, the study found that those who worked out with weights reduced their blood pressure and improved their overall coordination.

Yet, despite these tremendous physiological rewards, the biggest benefit of strength training may not be physical at all. What we're going to explore in this book is a shift in something far deeper and fundamental. It's about gaining a much greater power than a pumped-up bicep could ever provide. It's about rediscovering the essential relationship between your body and mind. In a manner of speaking, it's about using what I call "mindful movements" to learn how your body can help heal and strengthen your mind.

According to the National Institute of Mental Health, 18.8 million Americans suffer from depressive illness, 19 million have anxiety disorders, and 2 million are diagnosed with bipolar illness. Figures from the National Council on Alcoholism and Drug Dependence show that 18 million Americans have alcohol problems and 5 to 6 million have drug dependencies.

This book has been written for the millions of people who deal with emotional challenges of all kinds. Whether you are working to overcome depression or other mood disorders, suffer from too much stress, are in recovery from alcohol or drug abuse, or just want to feel more relaxed and physically stronger, this program is for you.

Exercise in the form of mindful movements is one of the best tools you can use to deal with any of these challenges. It can help you to achieve your highest level of inner and outer fitness.

Ultimately, it's about gaining control over your own life. I should know. I lost control of my life and was lucky enough to find my way back. In this book, I will tell you how I reclaimed myself and how you can too.

1

Exercise: My Downfall
and My Resurrection

Always bear in mind that your own resolution to succeed is more important than any other one thing.

⊷ Abraham Lincoln

I have a bumper sticker on my car. It says, "Another dope-less hope fiend."

It wasn't always that way. From age 12, when I took my first drink, until I became sober 17 years ago at age 22, I was hopelessly addicted to alcohol, drugs, and steroids. I was out of control. Like most addicts, I had to stare death in the face before I started the long road back to recovery.

It took a number of changes before I was ready. I had to face many uncomfortable truths about my past and about the way I had been conducting my life. Exercise was the one constant throughout my recovery. Once I put aside the "no pain, no gain" philosophy and focused on the psychological side of exercise, I began to heal my body and more importantly—my mind. That's why I want to share my story with you: to show you how strength training helped save my life.

I was 12 when I took my first drink. I hated the taste of the whiskey, which I stole from my grandfather's cabinet. But it made me feel like a new person. And I wanted to be a new person more than anything else in the world.

Life in my neighborhood of Randolph, Massachusetts, a suburb of Boston, looked like something right out of *Leave It to Beaver*. But it wasn't. I was short and small and had a speech impediment. I stuttered. As a result, I was the perfect foil for the older boys. I remember being excited about going away to camp one summer. My first day there, however, several of the older kids picked me up and put me into a half-filled trash dumpster and locked down the lid. The sad thing was, I didn't feel frightened, sitting there in that smelly dumpster. It seemed safer than my world on the outside.

In seventh grade, the same year I took up drinking seriously, I also began to lift weights. Drinking allowed me to escape the real world, which was full of pain and discouragement. The weights, I thought, would help me bulk up and become more popular with the girls. Both, in truth, were feeble attempts to mask the feelings of emptiness and self-doubt I felt inside.

During my senior year at Randolph High, I was lifting 225 pounds. I joined a health club and admired the body builders with huge muscles. It seemed to me that their bulk afforded them respect, something I craved. After a couple of weeks I learned their secret method of building muscle mass. It was dirty and illegal, but it worked. It was known around the gym as "d-bol," short for Dianabol, an anabolic steroid. As artificial growth hormones, steroids seemed to me to be the "breakfast of champions." I couldn't wait to try them.

My alcohol use progressed, as I preferred my vodka straight. I also began experimenting with cocaine and marijuana. Schoolwork became secondary to me. I got roaring drunk the night before I was to take the Scholastic Aptitude Test for college. Suffering from a raging hangover during the test, I just guessed at the answers. Not surprisingly, I did poorly.

My College Years Were No Different

I had to spend a semester at Fitchburg State in Central Massachusetts trying to pull my grades up before I was admitted to the University of Massachusetts at Amherst.

The summer following my freshman year I saved up enough money to get my fix of Dianabol. I wanted quick results so I started taking the pills right away. Within a few weeks, I had gained 20 pounds of muscle. It seemed like a dream come true. After that, I lost interest in nearly everything in my life except bulking up. I wanted to look like Mr. Olympia because I thought big biceps made me somebody. I had no idea of the nightmare that lay ahead. I was buying the dream now, and I would pay for it later. I had no clue about the size of the debt I was piling up. The sad truth was, though, even if I had known at that point, I wouldn't have cared.

By my senior year in college, I was hooked on alcohol and several street drugs, including cocaine, and six different types of steroids. I drifted through most of my classes, content to make D's, while most of my energy went into working out and partying. My workouts usually consisted of three-hour marathon sessions at the gym where I would lift the heaviest weights I could. I jerked the weights around in a frenzy to get bigger and bigger. I suffered a number of pulled muscles and small injuries working out this way. As a result, my workouts were erratic. Frustrated, I'd double my intake of alcohol and drugs during these down times. Physically, I may have been able to bench-press 400 pounds, but on the inside, I was a weakling.

Along the way, I suffered from what users call 'roid rages. A common side effect of steroids, it is a psychosis that leaves you in a perpetual state of anger. I became highly aggressive and always on edge. Combined with my constant drinking, I was a powder keg waiting to go off.

I was drunk or stoned the majority of the time in college. There were too many questions to answer when I was sober. Who was I? Where was I going? Did I have any value as a person? I didn't have the answers, so I numbed my feelings with alcohol, drugs, and extreme sessions of weightlifting.

In those days, my priority was not my classes, but where I would get my drugs. It didn't take me long to hear of a physician near the campus who would prescribe any steroid available—for a price, of course. I noticed that whenever I went into his office to get my prescription filled, his waiting room was filled with junkies of one type or another. The doctor shrugged and asked me what I wanted and in what quantity. Usually, I had to tell him how to spell the various types of steroids. After a while, he just handed me a prescription form and I filled it out myself. He also gave me needles so I could inject the drugs directly. So much for the Hippocratic Oath that physicians are supposed to abide by.

I usually had the prescriptions filled at a local pharmacy. Soon, I got to know the pharmacist. He stopped requiring a prescription and just sold me the steroids directly. My strength and muscle mass increased dramatically. They also made me very aggressive, and I experienced severe mood swings. But when I came off the steroids, which you must do from time to time, I lost strength and suffered from depression. When that happened, I compensated with even more drugs—including free-basing cocaine, speed, LSD, mushrooms, and pot—anything to keep from coming down. When I couldn't find any drugs, I binged on whiskey or tequila in order to escape from myself.

During my sophomore year, I went to Florida on spring break. To my horror, I realized I had left my drugs at home. Drunk, but anxious to find something stronger than alcohol, I encountered three men driving a low-slung car with darkened windows. One of them offered me some pills.

"Take these, man," he said. "They'll make you feel good."

I shrugged. Why not? I had no idea who the men were, where they came from, or what was in the pills, but I swallowed them with a chaser of vodka. They could have contained rat poison for all I knew, or cared. They turned out to be some sort of mild amphetamine. I survived the night, but the truth was I didn't much care.

Withdrawal and the Road Back

Somehow, early in December of 1987, I managed to graduate from the University of Massachusetts with a degree in economics. Because I had no idea what to do with my life, I planned on taking a couple of courses the following semester—and to party, party, party. The truth was I was petrified to go out into the real world.

Then something happened that changed my life.

During my last couple of years in college I had taken speech lessons to correct my stutter. My speech instructor, Adriana DiGrande, was an extremely positive person whom I came to greatly respect and admire. She was always kind and encouraging to me. I was shocked when, one afternoon during my winter break, she came to me with a frown on her face.

"Jeff, why don't you grow up?" she asked. "You need to go to a treatment center. You need to leave the drugs and alcohol behind. If you don't, you're going to die."

Her words had a tremendous effect on me. At that point in my life, I cared more about her opinion of me than anyone else's. That night, in the middle of a raucous New Year's Eve party, I made up my mind to quit everything cold turkey—the drugs, the alcohol, and the steroids. From time to time, I'd make some well-meaning promises to myself and quit the drugs and the booze for a few days. But no one can rationalize like a drunk, and before long, I'd be back on both again. This time I was more determined. I felt Adriana really cared for me as a person, and I wanted to show her I could do it.

At first, everything went well. I was living with my parents at the time, and I felt great. I seemed to have a tremendous amount of energy; so much, in fact, that I couldn't sleep at night. I thought the extra energy was terrific, but the fact was my body was going into shock. I had been a heavy user for nearly five years and going cold turkey was just too much for my system. I lost weight at an alarming rate, going from 185 to under 150 pounds in two months.

It all came crashing down one night when I found myself crawling around my room on my hands and knees, hallucinating and screaming. I thought rats were crawling out of my head. Hysterical, I tore at my hair. My father was horrified. He called the authorities, and an ambulance took me directly to the intensive care unit at a nearby hospital. I had an inflamed liver and my resting heart rate was 144 beats per minute—heart attack level. Miserable, I spent a month in the hospital and treatment center. Still withdrawing from the drugs and alcohol, I was hot one moment and freezing the next. I felt sick most of the time, and my attention span was about 15 seconds long. I was finally released a month later, physically weak and mentally exhausted.

Alcoholics Anonymous meetings and a long physical and mental rehabilitation followed. I stayed clean and sober. But even eight months later, I didn't feel whole. I was in terrible physical shape and felt lousy. I had kicked the street drugs, alcohol, and steroids, but I was depressed and listless. I stayed in bed much of the time. The only time I went out was to get ice cream and hot fudge. I had no ability to concentrate or otherwise function at all—not even to read a page in a magazine or watch television.

I ventured out to a gym one time, but it seemed the people who were working out had the same type of attitude that had gotten me into trouble in the first place. They were only interested in achieving huge muscles the fastest way they could. I was beyond that now. I knew the only meaningful workout was one in which I could begin to build myself from the inside out.

Exercise and a New Outlook

Months went by, and I began to stabilize. Knowing that I needed to improve all three of the critical elements in recovery—my emotional, my spiritual, and my physical well- being, I soon realized that the physical component was the missing piece. I began to wonder whether strength training might provide the answer. I bought some weights and began to carefully design a different type of workout. I became very keen on the connection between my mind and body. I hoped, by exploring that long-ignored relationship, I might be able to tap into a source of self-confidence.

When I began to exercise again I took a new attitude— I focused inward on how I felt, rather than outward on how I looked. My first step was to disregard the notion that to get strong you need to pump up the heaviest weights you can find. Instead, I began a program I call Mindful Movements. I began lifting lighter weights, slowly, with smooth, focused motions. At the same time, I began to concentrate on my breathing. This helped me relieve stress and get into a deep, rhythmic exercise. As I concentrated on moving each muscle, feeling each contraction and lengthening of the tissue, my workout became a form of meditation for me. I began to understand that the mind and body function together, like the flip sides to the same coin. As I worked out, I felt my mental attitude elevate a little more each day. My depression slowly dissipated, and I began to wake up each morning looking forward to the day. I was relaxed—primarily because I felt I was starting to take control.

This approach to weightlifting was making me feel whole again—and I looked forward to it for the right reasons. Lifting the lighter loads kept me from injury and burnout. I found great solace during the day in the thought that later I could retreat to my living room, which had become my make-shift gym, and begin my meditative workout. By now, "workout" had become an oxymoron for me. I was like a child with a wonderful new toy.

I was having fun!

The Power of Focused Exercise

Part of my experience was the excitement over the results. I could feel the tension drain away while I lifted. Each day, I felt my energy level grow. I felt more optimistic about my life and my future. My body gradually began to regain its former shape, but even more encouraging was the fact that I knew I was becoming spiritually and emotionally stronger.

Within months, I became so excited about the program and felt a passion to share it with others. This notion continued to grow until one summer's evening in 1990. I was helping a friend with his exercise program, and as we talked, he sensed that I was not satisfied with my day job. At the time, I was an accountant at a local bank. Our conversation went something like this:

"If you could do anything in the world," he asked, "what would it be?"

"I'd like to help teach people how to become whole again," I answered. "I'd like to show them the enormous potential of this program and how they can shape their minds as well as their muscles."

"Then do it," he said. "You won't be happy until you do."

I knew he was right.

The next day I quit the bank and started my company, Custom Fitness, in Quincy, Massachusetts. Later, I moved it to Boston. I created a safe, serene atmosphere that was the direct opposite of the competitive feeling that I had experienced in gyms. I knew this would be appealing to anyone who was in recovery as I was, or who was suffering from depression or any other kind of emotional challenge.

When I was coming off drugs and feeling lousy, I didn't want to go to a gym. At the time, most gyms were glitzy and espoused the no pain, no gain philosophy. This is still true today. In other words, people think that for some reason, exercise has to be painful or difficult to be beneficial. And at most gyms, trainers and members alike are primarily focused on how they look on the outside instead of how they are feeling on the inside.

Today, as in 1990, when I started Custom Fitness, I take a sensitive approach to my clients' feelings and needs and employ trainers who understand this method. We create a program that is appropriate for each individual, and gently and carefully guide each person through. We help him or her focus on each movement and concentrate on each working muscle.

My primary goal with this program is to relieve stress and help people feel better. I want everyone to experience the psychological benefits and change their perception of exercise. In fact, my clients who suffer from depression make sure to keep their appointments because they know they will feel better when they're finished. Feeling better comes first; physical changes, while important, come second. Still, after they begin exercising, many of my clients are faced with an exciting task—purchasing a new wardrobe to complement their new shape!

Today, I'm lucky enough to be working with scores of clients from all over the world who are intrigued by this new approach to mind-body fitness. Most are suffering from some degree of depression or other emotional difficulties, or are in recovery from substance abuse. Others want to work off everyday stress and establish a fitness program that's right for them.

The goal of these workouts isn't to look like a supermodel or Mr. America. It's something far more important and long-lasting than that. It is more like learning how to conduct an orchestra. The emphasis is on how to blend your body and mind into movements of perfect harmony. And when this happens, when you can feel your body moving, when you can feel your muscles as they stretch and grow, an amazing realization takes place—that you are fully alive and strong.

For years I had been abusing substances because I felt that I had little self-worth. Worse, I felt I had little control over my life. I took drugs in part because I felt so powerless. But now that's all changed. I know now what incredible machines our minds and bodies are, and how, by tuning them to a fine harmony, by orchestrating thought and action, we can empower them both.

Gaining that power was an enormous stress release for me. More importantly, it gave me back control over my body, my mind, and my life.

It Can Do the Same for You

In Chapter 2, I show, in more depth, how exercise can make you feel better emotionally. In Chapter 3, several of my clients tell what exercise has done for them. In Chapter 4, we talk about nutrition and your mood. In Chapter 5, I talk more about my philosophy of exercise. Chapters 6 through 9 give you exercise programs that you can easily do at home.

Let's get started.

2

Exercise, Wellness, and Your Moods

*Iron rusts from disuse, water loses its purity from stag-
nation...even so does inaction sap the vigors of the
mind. Did I exercise my mind today?*

  ❧ Leonardo da Vinci

As I have told you, I was once a mental and physical time
bomb.

In my late teens and early twenties, there were times
when I was taking up to six steroids, as well as alcohol,
cocaine, and other drugs to balance the effects of the steroids. I was suffering as a result. When I quit cold turkey, my
resting heart rate, 144 beats per minute, was more than
twice what it should have been and lingered in the heart
attack danger zone. My liver was a mess. My weight had
dropped from 185 pounds to under 150 pounds.

I had used harsh exercise and dangerous drugs to build
up a body that looked strong, but in reality was weakening
from the stress and the poison. Mentally and emotionally I
was wounded, lost, and losing ground. For about a year after

I got off the drugs, I lay listless, not knowing what to do. While I was no longer abusing drugs and alcohol, a deep depression set in.

But in time, something amazing began to happen. I began to find myself drawn to exercise for the right reasons, and it helped me find my way back.

While I had been over-exercising and taking drugs to cut myself off from the pain I was feeling, I began to use gentle, meditative doses of regular exercise to reconnect with who I was, for better or worse, and to build my self-esteem. Doing something that was good for me—increasing my physical strength—was self-affirming. Weight training became a tool I used to build emotional strength for coping with life.

I began to discover what real wellness is—not only the absence of illness, but also the condition of good physical and mental health that we can all strive for and maintain with exercise, proper diet, and good sleep habits.

During this process, I found my mission in life: to help others with challenges like mine find their way to wellness through exercise—and the greater inner strength and peace that comes with it. This was a dramatic reversal for me. My hope is that exercise can lead to a dramatic reversal for you—if that is what is needed.

Proven by Research

As it turns out, I stumbled onto something very important, so important that scientists around the country have been studying it for years: the effect of exercise on mood and quality of life.

Why is exercise so powerful? While research continues, and we don't have all the answers quite yet, we have some good ideas as to why. "There is a consensus that exercise is intrinsically beneficial. It acts as an antidepressant and lowers anxiety," explains Alex Vuckovic, M.D., assistant clinical professor of psychiatry at Harvard Medical School, and medical director of the Pavilion at McLean Hospital in Belmont, Massachusetts.

"It is fair to suggest that, for reasons not yet understood, physical activity releases chemicals in the brain, neurotransmitters which mimic the qualities of the opiate drugs that we use in medicine to relieve pain," he explains. "This class of chemicals, when released, appears to enhance feelings of well-being. That's the theoretical basis for some of these findings."

The 1996 Surgeon General's *Report on Physical Activity and Health*, which analyzed all of the research findings that had been completed regarding the effects of exercise on mental and physical health concluded:

Physical activity appears to relieve symptoms of depression and anxiety and improve mood. Regular physical activity may reduce the risk of developing depression, although further research is needed on this topic...Physical activity appears to improve health-related quality of life by enhancing psychological well-being and by improving physical functioning in persons compromised by poor health.

The report also clearly states that weight training, in particular, is important to health:

> Recent recommendations from experts also suggest that cardio-respiratory endurance activity should be supplemented with strength-developing exercises at least twice per week for adults, in order to improve musculoskeletal health, maintain independence in performing the activities of daily life, and reduce the risk of falling.

It recommends that people start slowly, just as I do:

> Most musculoskeletal injuries related to physical activity are believed to be preventable by gradually working up to a desired level of activity and by avoiding excessive amounts of activity.

Improving Your Life Day to Day

Practically speaking, what does this mean to you? How do these general conclusions translate to your life each day? Here is what exercise can do for you when pursued regularly and with the proper attitude:

+ It releases brain chemicals that can elevate your mood. When you weight train, you are subtly injuring your muscles—a good thing. Muscle development occurs during the repair of those microscopic injuries. To reduce any minor physical discomfort that may be associated with this process, your central nervous system signals your brain to release a class of chemicals—endorphins and enkephalins—that mask pain while enhancing your mood.

+ A session of exercise may relieve your anxiety and raise your energy level, all of which can lift your spirits. You may feel these positive effects for several hours afterward.

+ It can give you a sense of control. Exercise really is about acquiring a skill. Learning something different and healthy can give you a sense of mastery, the pride in feeling that you've accomplished something new.

+ It can encourage you to improve your wellness in other ways. This increased sense of control, this positive momentum you feel, may make changing other habits easier. For example, you may be less apt to eat junk food when you are doing something that is beneficial for your health and well-being. And you may be more likely to quit smoking if that has been a problem.

+ It may distract you from problems and negative feelings. Strength training may help you "burn off" and let go of any destructive thoughts that you may be harboring. In addition, just the fact that you are improving your health may improve your mood.

+ It improves your body image. There is a link between exercise and self-esteem. Being in better physical condition creates a more positive body image. That is, you look in the mirror and you like seeing your body fat decreasing and your physique becoming more tightened and toned. You will also notice an improvement in strength, balance, and flexibility—all of which feels just great.

✦ It improves your overall health. Exercise can reduce lower back pain, which can bring you tremendous relief. You will experience improved lung and heart function, which will not only safeguard your health long-term but also make daily tasks easier to accomplish. You may also enjoy knowing that exercise can lower your blood pressure, induce positive changes in your blood cholesterol, and strengthen your bones.

✦ It helps prevent relapse. According to the National Mental Health Association, exercise plays an important part in the successful treatment of a variety of mental illnesses. It states, "People who have major depression and anxiety disorders are significantly (60 percent) less likely to relapse if they exercise regularly and continue exercising over time than if they take medication alone."

An Important Part of Treatment

As a result, a growing number of physicians are prescribing exercise to their patients, including those who are stressed, going through difficult times, recovering from alcohol and substance abuse, or are suffering from mood disorders. Dr. Vuckovic is one such physician.

"There have been studies that show the beneficial effect of exercise in treating milder forms of depression and that exercise can enhance the benefits of psychotherapy and medication as part of an overall treatment plan," he explains. "As a result, I absolutely do prescribe exercise for my patients. People with depression may not be motivated to exercise, which may lead to weight gain and a sedentary lifestyle. People with anxiety may be so preoccupied with stresses that come at them day to day; they may not take time for themselves. Exercise is an important part of a treatment plan in both cases."

Dr. Vuckovic further points out that exercise also helps to counter some of the side effects his patients experience as part of their treatment.

"The more in tune my patients are with the need for making lifestyle changes when they become stressed, the more exercise can empower them to take control of it," he continues. "Whenever I do an evaluation with a patient, I try to determine how and if exercise plays a role in his or her lifestyle. Fitness can help my patients offset some of the negative elements caused by their illness or course of treatment. Some medications cause weight gain, and I emphasize that it is vital for patients to keep themselves fit."

What About Your Local Gym

Exercise programs abound. You see gyms advertised all the time on television and in your local paper. What's wrong with them? Nothing, if they work for you. If they do, I'd encourage you to sign up at the facility of your choice. I certainly would never discourage anyone from doing that, if it feels right.

A common problem with many of these gyms is that they emphasize the quick fix—fast weight loss or rock-hard abs. Most completely overlook the psychological benefits of exercise, and that's a shame.

In addition, they tend to give people little or no attention. If they do provide instruction, the trainers often expect too much too fast. They've simply forgotten what it's like to be new to exercise. It takes tremendous sensitivity to help people get started, and most trainers in gyms don't have that touch. Unfortunately, as a result, people sometimes find themselves feeling frustrated and drop out.

Instead, the program in this book emphasizes a slower, gentler, more individualized program that emphasizes the mind as well as the body, which Dr. Vuckovic agrees is important.

"Clearly, the more individualized the program it is, the more it can be shaped to fit a person's needs and take advantage of the therapeutic power of exercise," he says. "People may fear how they look, so getting themselves out there to exercise is difficult. As a result, they may be poorly served by institutional programs that put them with other people. A realistic and specialized approach is important for these individuals. Rather than emphasizing the need to get buff, this program begins with getting the mind and body together. In that way, this program is far ahead of the game."

You can do this program in the privacy of your own home. When I put this together, I considered the many struggles that people have with exercise—that many of my clients have and that I once had myself. I've created this book to help people get over the barriers they may face when starting an exercise program. I encourage you to start at your own pace, in the way that makes you the most comfortable.

Getting It Done

Still, creating an exercise habit in your life will take some self-management.

I realize that doing this can be a challenge if you're feeling depressed and the thought of just moving is hard. Or if the details of everyday life seem to overwhelm you because you're feeling anxious or your schedule is tremendously hectic. Or you feel just plain lousy because you're in recovery.

Sometimes you just won't feel like exercising. It's that simple.

Still, I'm going to give you some straight talk so you can discipline yourself when needed. But I'm also going to tell you to go easy on yourself. This program is supposed to be gentle and in no way extreme. My best advice:

+ Schedule exercise sessions. As with other appointments in your life, it is important to set aside times for your exercise sessions. Block off 40 minutes, three days a week. Write these down in your appointment book or Palm Pilot. Unlike a dentist visit, you will be looking forward to this.
+ Eat a light, healthy snack an hour before you exercise. Even gentle exercise takes energy. If you're too hungry, you may feel tired, or may choose eating instead of exercise.

✤ Don't let yourself contemplate too long whether or not to exercise. You may talk yourself out of it. Instead, make that move to get started. I promise you'll feel 100 percent better when you are done.

✤ Plan to do as much as you can. If you do at least a little exercise several times a week, you'll find it much easier to stick with the program. Consistency is the key. You'll be surprised: once you build the habit, you'll begin to look forward to your next exercise session.

✤ If you're having a bad day and don't feel like exercising, lighten it up. Tell yourself you'll do one-half, or even one-quarter of the exercises. Don't let yourself feel bad; give yourself credit for having done something. The last thing you want to do is have guilty feelings about exercise. The idea is to lower the mental barrier that you're feeling and do what you can.

✤ Reward yourself for what you've accomplished. Think of doing something for yourself that is both healthy and meaningful. Something that really does make you feel good; maybe get a massage or enjoy a day at the spa. This is important because you want to create positive reinforcement for yourself. Besides, you deserve it.

The overall message here: exercise can make a tremendous difference in your emotional wellness. Use this program to get started toward making a gentle program of regular physical activity part of your lifestyle. Use it as a tool to conquer the challenges you face, whatever they are, and enjoy the best life that you can have. You owe it to yourself.

3

Gaining Control: Stories from the Front

I thank God for my handicaps, for, through them, I have found myself, my work, and my spirituality.

✧ Helen Keller

It has been one of the true joys of my life to watch people respond to and find success with this program. Just as I have.

My clients run the gamut; they are a diverse group of individuals with various backgrounds and occupations. Some suffer from mental illness such as depression, anxiety disorder, or bipolar illness. While others face physical challenges, many are dealing with everyday stress, are burned out, have low self-esteem and are struggling to find a way to cope with modern pressures.

I've seen people grieve over the loss of a loved one, from the loss of a job, or go through a painful divorce. Some of my clients have overcome physical difficulties, or have lost the extra weight they've struggled with for years and have finally kept it off. Often times, I've been a witness as people find a renewed sense of their lives by making exercise a part of their recovery from alcohol or drug abuse.

During the many years that I have used this approach to exercise, I have seen some real, life-altering changes in the people I've worked with. The transitions that many of my clients have experienced have been dramatic in many cases, just as the transition that I've made has been dramatic.

In this chapter, I'd like to relate some of these success stories in the hope that you will relate to them. To protect the identity of my clients, you should know that I have changed the names and the circumstances I describe. But the essence of each anecdote is true.

George: For Physical Strength and Balance

One client I've worked with for many years is 47-year-old George, who was born with a birth defect, which caused a muscle imbalance. I met him when I was working out at a local gym. George's handicap was obvious; his right leg dragged quite a bit as he walked. And when he lifted weights, one side of the barbell went up faster and more easily than the other.

Prior to taking on George as a client I observed him working out with another fellow, Tim, who was obviously in it for his ego. It was clear to me that Tim was overly focused on the amount of weight he could lift. He'd load up the bar with 200 pounds and bring it back down three or four inches, obviously not going through a full range of motion. I noticed his back came up off the weight bench (not good), and he'd grimace and groan like he was Superman (really dumb). He would then high-five the other guys as if he had really accomplished something (wrong).

The truth is, Tim was using completely improper form that wasn't going to give him the results he wanted and was likely to injure him. It was obvious to me from his pear-shaped body that he was getting little benefit—if any at all—from his time spent in the gym. Tim was completely wasting his time, and would have been better off spending those two hours doing something else. He and his buddy Joe, who lifted in much the same way, were poster children for macho weightlifters, the type of guys who wear torn t-shirts to show off their physiques and brag to women at bars about how much they are lifting at the gym. They were the stereotypical weightlifters.

I mention Tim and Joe because they were having a very poor influence on George. Working out with them was actually making his muscle imbalance worse. But, fortunately, George saw me working out, and we started talking. We established a relationship, and soon I began to train him.

I clearly stated to George that lifting heavy weight was neither important nor healthy; rather it was better to lift the amount of weight that was appropriate for his abilities, using proper form. In the end, doing this is what made George successful. While he had trouble walking before, George walks with little difficulty now. Our sessions have increased the strength in his body and given him a new confidence and sense of his abilities. "I feel a lot more whole," he once told me. That feeling is clearly reflected in his bearing when he walks now and by the smile on his face.

You can believe that hearing these words from George made me smile then and still does now.

Arthur: For Emotional Balance

My client Arthur, who is 62 and a very successful entrepreneur, has a tendency to overwork, sometimes to the point of near exhaustion. "While I was very successful in my professional life, I had little or no personal life," he remembers. "My entire life revolved around my company. As a result, my moods rode the roller coaster along with my business. I knew that I needed help, and this program is part of that help. For the first time in my life, I'm learning that less really is more. Before, I thought the answer was always to try harder. But what I was doing was breaking myself down. Now I've learned how to build myself up."

The slow, highly focused exercises in this program have shown Arthur that you can build real strength gradually and easily— and be relaxed while doing it. "I feel that I'm getting stronger physically and emotionally all the time. For the first time, I have some balance in my life—and I like it."

Susan: To Combat Stress and Regain Energy

Susan is a Boston-based physician, another over-achiever whose high stress level left her constantly unhappy and frustrated and on the verge of quitting her job. She also felt guilty, fearing that she may not be giving her patients the care and attention they needed. As a result, she was continually questioning most of the major decisions that she had made in her life.

As a physician, it was very hard for Susan to admit that she, herself, needed help. However, she decided to see a psychologist who concluded that Susan was not only suffering from stress from overwork but from depression as well. Susan was surprised when her psychologist referred her to me. We worked together for six months on a strength training program. In the process, Susan learned to slow down and relax more. She not only recovered her former high level of energy but also gained a new level of self-confidence. It was based on the notion that when she controlled her body, she could also manage her stress level, a major revelation that has changed her attitude. She now feels happier and much more competent in her job.

Sarah: For Emotional Healing

Other people I've known have used this exercise program as an aid to emotional healing from painful experiences.

Sarah came to me five years ago after hearing about me from a friend. Sarah was at wit's end; she had just ended her second marriage and was going through the stressful, sad rigors of a painful divorce. She found that her husband had been unfaithful, and she was devastated. "When I came to you, I was feeling so lost. I never thought that I'd feel any kind of happiness again," she told me recently.

But over time, I have seen Sarah undergo a tremendous change. She has regained control over her life, choosing to enter a completely new career. "The stronger I began to feel physically, the stronger I began to feel mentally. I realized that, despite the choices I had made, despite the choices my former husband had made, there was a future, and it was mine. I've always had a knack for interior decorating, so I decided to take some courses. Eventually, I finished a degree, and now I work in a field I love. But I always make time for exercise, because it has become a cornerstone in my life."

Bob: For Healthy Weight Loss

Weight loss is a big issue with many people these days, and so it was with Bob, who came to me four years ago. At the age of 30, Bob was 75 pounds overweight. He told me he wanted to succeed and lose the weight once and for all. While his father had suggested that Bob find a personal trainer, he hesitated at first. The personal trainers he had heard of seemed too tough, almost like track coaches.

"I'd always hated gym class and sports in high school, so the idea of going to a personal trainer wasn't at all appealing to me," Bob told me. "While I did compete as an athlete, it was always too competitive and too painful for me." With that in mind, I asked Bob to come in three times a week for my gentle program, and I let him show me the amount of exercise that was most comfortable for him. "I don't feel any pressure and really enjoy doing the workout. I'm not competing against anyone, not even myself. I feel so great that I've lost the weight and have kept it off."

Fran: To Manage a Cluster of Challenges

Like millions of other Americans, 35-year-old Fran suffers from bipolar illness. She has, at times, been hospitalized for her illness. Now, she continues intensive therapy. Fran also carries some extra weight. Due to the fact that she has trouble with her thyroid, she takes medication for her illness and has a tendency to binge on food. When she came to me, Fran weighed 200 pounds. She lost 30 pounds in the first 6 months and has kept it off.

"I've been struggling with my weight for several years now. I'd take 20 pounds off, and in no time, put it right back on. When I started a new medication recently, I looked around for other things that would help me. I realized that I needed to get into a fitness program. Getting fit had helped me in the past. I thought of getting a personal trainer, but I wanted to find someone who would understand what I was dealing with. I didn't want to go into an intimidating club."

Fran has regained what we call functional fitness—the ability to do the tasks of life safely and easily. "The exercise program has done me a lot of good. Before, it was hard for me just to get around. Now, I can get out of a car without huffing and puffing. I'm strong enough to go on a walk."

While Fran does have a fitness center in her apartment building that she could use, she feels that she needs the support she gets from this program.

"There is a real acceptance of who you are here. Sometimes, when I'm having a real bad day, I just do a few minutes—all that I can handle. I've learned exercises that I can do at home with exercise bands. I also try to walk an hour once a week. If I can do these things, I can do other things. If there is something I can do that will help me feel more positive, I need to do it."

Allie: A Big Part of Her Overall Treatment Program

One client who was referred to me by her psychiatrist is 40-year-old Allie, who started this program in January of last year. She told me that she had been treated for depression since the age of 16, taking a variety of medications as part of her treatment program. Allie had been trying to exercise on and off for 10 years, believing that it would help relieve her symptoms of depression.

Early on, it became clear to me that Allie was making a supreme effort to come see me. Just before our first session was to begin, she called, telling me that she could not find her way. She was almost in tears, and I told her it was okay. When she finally arrived an hour later, we began to talk. I heard such pain in her voice and saw it in her body language. It brought me back to my feeling of utter hopelessness when I first came off of alcohol and drugs. After talking with her, I actually experienced some flashbacks of my living hell so many years ago.

Knowing that this program could make a big difference in her life, I was determined to help Allie feel better, as I had come to feel better. She told me that she had tried several antidepressants, but none had seemed to work for her. Her psychiatrist, one of the best in the field, had prescribed a drug that often made her feel sluggish and tired.

As we talked, I heard more about her family history. She told me that her father was the owner of several health clubs in California. Allie had worked out in the past, but it was always with the no pain, no gain mentality. She got this from her father, who would always pressure her into exercising until exhaustion. Understandably, she was a bit turned off from exercising. I emphasized to her that this program is not like that at all. I explained to her that more is not always better. You do not have to suffer through a three-hour exercise program and feel soreness and exhaustion later to get the results you want. Actually, that approach is counter-productive.

Allie had to put her past experience with exercise behind her, and fortunately, she's been able to do that. "I've never been able to sustain a program," she told me. "I'd join a gym and take classes, go for a while, but then I'd slack off. But, knock on wood, this program seems to be working. It's a big thing for me to have structure and accountability, and so far, I've kept it going."

Allie comes in three times a week for an hour. We'll do some abdominal work, and then use the leg machines. Next, we may do some chest exercises; some back work, and finally some shoulder and arm exercises. Then, to strengthen her heart and lungs, she may use the elliptical trainer or the exercise bicycle for 20 or 25 minutes, depending on how much energy she has on a particular day.

"There are days when just moving is hard for me. But I know that this is something that I have to do, so I just do it," Allie says. "Afterward, I'm glad that I've done it. I definitely plan to continue. I don't see any reason to not do it. It's the only thing, exercise-wise, that I've ever been able to maintain."

My hope for you is that you will enjoy similar success and this program will help you gain control over the issues that are important to you in your life.

4

Your Diet and Your Mood

We are what we repeatedly do. Excellence then is not an act, but a habit.

    ∾ Aristotle

When I got off the drugs and alcohol, it was a good thing. No question. But, in time, I realized that I had much more work to do in other areas of my life. Before I could feel good, really good, I had to improve my eating habits.

For example, I began in the morning, going wild on coffee loaded with sugar, drinking up to three pots throughout the day. For dinner, I'd often head to McDonald's for a Big Mac Extra Value Meal®, which includes super-sized fries and Coca-Cola®. Or I'd buy boxes of those fat-free cookies and cakes that were loaded with sugar. At night, I'd find myself overeating to mask my negative feelings. Then I would starve myself the next day out of guilt. But by evening, I'd feel too hungry and overeat again. While it was good that I was no longer using, I was caught in a tough negative cycle. In some ways, I was still out of control.

I can laugh now, imagining my face covered with cookie and cake crumbs, and my car littered with fast-food wrappers.

On one hand, I was very much on the right track, going through therapy and attending 12-step meetings regularly. However, I found some flaws in the system. While I respect and applaud much about these programs, I saw people drinking too much coffee, feasting on sugar-laden donuts, and smoking cigarette after cigarette at the meetings.

I realized that I needed to treat myself better than that to fully recover. What I had to do was stop substituting food and caffeine for drugs. While I had taken 12 steps forward in my recovery, it was as if I was taking 12 backwards when I overindulged on fat-free cakes, french fries, and sugar-loaded coffee.

Gradually, one positive choice, healthy exercise, helped me make another positive choice in my life, a healthy diet. As I changed my diet, I began to feel more positive, energized, and much more in control.

Does this sound familiar to you? If it does, don't feel guilty or embarrassed as I did. Instead, be kind enough to yourself, and take a good look at your diet. Make sure you are eating in a way that is good for both your mind and body. The food you eat plays a major role in your physical and emotional health.

Please consider the suggestions in this chapter, many of which come from Amy Gleason, M.S., R.D., a senior nutritionist at McLean Hospital in Belmont, Massachusetts.

Cut Caffeine Consumption

While one cup of coffee may make you feel more alert, increasing your physical and mental performance, larger quantities can cause anxiety, fatigue, dizziness, irritability, and sleeplessness. Many of these symptoms stem from a drop in blood sugar. Black coffee alone can cause these symptoms. When coffee is loaded with sugar, it can greatly exaggerate them and really rock your moods. You may feel a rush of energy, followed by a sudden drop within about an hour. Sugar-loaded, caffeinated soft drinks may affect you in the same way.

"I highly recommend that people stay away from caffeine, if possible, in particular, caffeine with sugar," says Gleason. "What you get is an initial spiking of blood sugar, followed by a sudden drop. Caffeine can also disrupt your sleep. Being sleep deprived can affect your ability to cope during the day. In addition, if your sleep is disrupted, you may feel tempted to get up and eat, which will add extra weight."

If you have been drinking multiple cups of coffee or cans of soda daily and want to cut back, Gleason recommends doing it gradually. Caffeine is a drug; quitting cold turkey is not recommended. If you do, you may experience headaches as a sign of withdrawal. They can be severe.

"I'd taper slowly, cutting out one cup of coffee every three to seven days. You also might want to do it when you don't have a lot going on, such as when you're on vacation, so you can give yourself time to adjust," she suggests.

What if you're on medications that make you feel drowsy? In that case, I understand the temptation to drink coffee. But it would be better to take a walk or drink some water instead," Gleason says.

Eat Your Breakfast and Don't Forget Your Protein

People who don't care much for breakfast tend to skip it and fill their stomachs with coffee. Others choose sugary foods in an effort to get themselves going. If that's your habit, consider how you are robbing yourself of needed energy. As we said, although you'll get an initial rush from coffee and sugar, your blood sugar will drop rapidly, so you're really starting your day at quite a deficit.

Instead, it's better to eat a small breakfast of fruit or plain yogurt. Avoid unnecessary sugar by adding your own fresh or frozen fruit instead of buying the flavored variety of yogurt. Or choose whole grain cereals made of wheat bran, barley, or oats. If you like toast, try whole wheat instead of white bread. What you don't want to do is load it with butter and sweetened jams; try cottage cheese or natural peanut butter for a change. Don't forget eggs; eaten in moderation, they are a great choice. "They're good because they contain choline, which may benefit your memory," Gleason says.

"It's also a good idea to have some sort of protein in the morning, along with a complex carbohydrate. If you do, your mood and your energy level will remain stable longer. If you eat a sugary muffin early in the morning, you'll feel tired by mid-morning, and you will be more likely to crave sweets all day long."

For other meals, you'll also want to choose some good lean meats such as turkey breast, extra lean hamburger, lean cuts of pork, fish, canned tuna packed in water rather than oil, and skinless chicken. Protein contains all-important amino acids that your body needs. Include protein in your diet, and you won't find yourself hungry as often.

"Protein-rich foods also help your body make tryptophan, which is a precursor to serotonin, a chemical in the brain which affects your mood," Gleason says.

What if meat is not your thing? Then be sure to eat adequate amounts of beans and tofu for the protein they contain.

Eat Small Meals Often

Are you, like a lot of people, programmed to eat two or three larger meals per day? Or do you have a tendency to starve yourself during the day and eat one extra-large meal at night, thinking that you're going to lose weight?

Whether you realize it or not, habits like these can also affect your moods, your energy level, and your ability to stick with a healthy diet.

Rather than eating at arbitrary times—morning, noon and night whether you're hungry or not—Gleason says it's better to eat five or six smaller meals, timed to coincide with your real hunger. Doing so is more likely to keep your blood sugar at a more even level throughout the day, which should help keep your moods more stable.

The key is to combine foods made of complex carbohydrates such as fruits, vegetables, beans and whole grain breads

with foods made of protein and some fat such as peanut butter, nuts and avocados. Healthy fats provide a relatively lon-
ger-term energy supply, and complex carbohydrates provide a
shorter-term energy supply.

"I recommend that people eat these foods every three to
four hours to keep their energy level up. Eating these food
combinations often throughout the day will help prevent
spikes in blood sugar," says Gleason.

Once again, you want to stay away from excessive
amounts of simple, processed carbohydrates, such as white
bread, pasta, candy, cookies, and pastries. Since these foods
have been processed and lack the fiber that slows down
absorption, they are digested and released quickly into the
bloodstream. You get a spike of insulin in your blood, which
sends your blood sugar level down. This can have a negative
affect on your mood. Soon, you're hungry again. You may
experience cravings and feel like binge eating. Also, if your
insulin level is high, you will be more likely to store extra
energy as fat.

Complex carbohydrates such as fruits, vegetables, and
whole grains are digested more slowly and have a more gradual affect on your blood sugar. If you like pasta and rice, go for
it. Just choose whole grain pasta and brown rice. They also
contain important vitamins and fiber, which are healthier.

"In addition, if you're tempted to substitute the artificial
sweetener Aspartame for sugar, don't do it," Gleason warns.
"Aspartame decreases tryptophan, the substance the body
needs to produce serotonin, which affects mood."

If you do eat small meals more often, as Gleason recommends, you won't feel starved, and as a result, you'll make better food choices. Whenever you're too hungry, you're more likely to eat junk food because it's convenient and you can't wait for something healthier.

"While these changes are important, make them gradually, so you don't get frustrated," Gleason advises. "If you try to change your eating habits all at once, it can be overwhelming. To be successful, concentrate on changing your meal structure first, before you change the type of food you eat."

Be Finicky About Fats

It's helpful to understand one thing: a certain amount of the right fats is important to your diet, as fat is needed for your body to absorb fat-soluble vitamins, such as A, D, E, and K. Fat is also important to brain function. However, it is important to choose the right fats to protect your health.

Generally speaking, you'll want to choose monounsaturated fats such as olives, most nuts, peanut butter, olive and canola oil, as well as polyunsaturated fats such as safflower, soybean, and cottonseed oils. Stay away from saturated fats. These are found in animal products such as butter, cheese, whole milk, ice cream, cream, and fatty meats. They are also found in some vegetable oils: coconut, palm, and palm kernel oils. You'll also want to avoid trans fats, which are formed when vegetable oils are processed to become solid. Trans fats are found in fried foods, commercial baked goods (such as donuts, cookies, and crackers), processed foods, margarine, and other foods. Like saturated fats, trans fats can clog your arteries.

While trans fats and saturated fat can raise the level of LDL, or bad cholesterol, in your blood, vegetable-based fats can raise the level of HDL, or good cholesterol.

At this moment, package labels do not highlight the amount of trans fat in processed foods. To identify them, just look at the ingredients on the package for the word hydrogenated.

"In addition, people with bipolar disorder and depression may want to include dark fishes, such as salmon, tuna, mackerel, and blue fish in their diets two or three times a week. These foods contain omega-3 fatty acids, which have been shown to benefit people with these disorders. If you don't like fish, I'd suggest getting these oils in the form of capsules," Gleason says.

Be Safe with Supplements

If you eat a balanced diet, chances are you will be getting the necessary amounts of nutrients for general health. But if you find that there are some food groups that you just can't eat, and you have a sense that your diet is not completely balanced, you may want to consider taking a vitamin supplement.

However, this is another case when more is not necessarily better, so it's best to stick with the recommended dosage on the package label.

"Generally, I suggest that people take Vitamins E, C, and B-complex," says Gleason. "A daily multivitamin with minerals may be fine. If you're over 55, I suggest a B-complex because it has the essential B vitamins which are good for energy production, memory, and brain function."

"Finally, if you are taking antidepressant medication, you will want to stay away from herbal supplements, which may interfere with some antidepressants. Generally speaking, if you are on medication, it makes sense to check with your doctor before taking vitamins, or supplements of any kind," says Gleason.

Enjoy a Pre-Exercise Snack

Believe it or not, one dependable way to stay with your exercise program is to eat one of your small meals about an hour beforehand. If you don't, you may experience a drop in blood sugar, and as a result, you may feel too tired to exercise.

The good news is this snack doesn't have to be complicated. It can consist of an apple, yogurt, banana, fruit juice, or other healthy foods that you can carry with you. Be watchful, however, when it comes to granola bars or other processed foods, as they tend to be loaded with sugar.

"If you do eat before you exercise, you'll have a more effective session, and you won't feel light-headed in the middle of it," Gleason says. "Just be sure that you don't eat something bulky that will make your stomach feel uncomfortable. And be sure to drink plenty of water. If you're dehydrated, you may feel sluggish. Generally speaking, it's a good idea to carry a refillable water bottle, not only to your exercise session, but with you all day."

Exercise to Sleep and Eat Well

Regular exercise can make the changes we describe here a lot easier. For starters, it helps reduce stress and the eating associated with it.

Exercise can also help you sleep well. As you let go of your stress and negative feelings through exercise, falling asleep will be easier. If you wake up well-rested, you'll be less likely to rely on coffee and sugar—and get into the negative blood-sugar cycle that we've discussed.

If you cut back on coffee, caffeine will not disrupt your sleep. A good night's sleep can help you "eat healthy" throughout the day. You will then be less likely to mistake fatigue for hunger, and eat when you don't need to. You will also be less likely to make impulsive food choices when you do need to eat.

When I became sober, exercise helped me turn my eating and other negative lifestyle habits around. It can do that for you, too.

5

My Philosophy of Exercise: Mindful Movements

Slow motion gets you there faster.

ॐ Anonymous

When it comes to this program, I'd like to assure you of two things: one, it is going to be different from any that you have done or even heard of before; two, you can count on enjoying it. Remember, its main goal is to relieve stress and help you feel better, but you'll also get the added bonus of a toned physique.

No doubt, these are different notions for you, whether you are a non-exerciser or have had prior experience at a gym or with exercise videos. There were probably times when you tried and gave up on exercise. Perhaps you became sore from working out too hard, didn't know the correct technique and ended up hurting yourself, or felt intimidated by the buff bodies at the gym.

In the past, the thought of exercising may have created added anxiety. That will not happen with this program.

Having had the no pain, no gain workout mentality, I felt if I wasn't exercising to exhaustion, then I wasn't doing myself any good. I've learned that grueling workouts are not beneficial and in fact end up hurting. Since the eighth grade I had been exercising with the wrong approach. I would spend as long as two or three hours lifting as much weight as possible. It left me worn out afterwards and it was no fun, really. Often, I would injure myself, straining muscles and ligaments and even chipping bones. When I gave up that philosophy my transformation began.

Numbness is the only way to describe my mental and physical state when I began my recovery from years of substance abuse. My mind and body had been shut off from one another, and I felt there was no hope that my life would get any better. I realized that I could no longer bench-press 400 pounds, and that was somewhat depressing to me.

Still, I really wanted to get back into exercising, so I decided that I had to change my way of thinking. I began to focus more on the movement during each exercise. This would put me in a nearly trance-like and relaxed state. Over time, the results I achieved amazed me.

Exercise Became Meditation

Exercise in this way became a meditative experience for me; it not only awakened my body, but more importantly, it awakened my mind. There is such a strong mind-body connection through strength training when it is done correctly and with the proper attitude.

Instead of curling 150 pounds, I started off with 30 pounds, focusing completely on my biceps, feeling the contraction and tightening in the muscles of my upper arms. As I lowered the weight, I would feel every fiber in my biceps stretching and opening. By focusing on these movements, I tuned into my body's power and strength. Doing so not only awakened my body but made me feel more alive emotionally.

When I was using heavy weights, there was no way I could focus on the working muscles. I had to think about lifting the weight any way possible. Otherwise, I might find myself pinned underneath hundreds of pounds.

I found that it is much better to use light to moderate weights because you can keep your mind on the movement, and you don't have to be so concerned about safety. It may take some time to get that mind-body connection going, but once you do, you will want to continue; there is nothing else like it.

Anyone, young or old, male or female, will be able to adapt this program to fit his or her life. I've made sure of that. I don't like to call this a workout program, because this is not a form of hard physical labor as many other exercise programs are. My goal for people is to release stress and feel better.

In this chapter, I will describe the benefits of this program, the simple equipment required, and some tips to keep in mind as you begin. We will describe, in the next four chapters, the specific way to perform each exercise.

Proper breathing techniques will be discussed as part of the overall goal of stress-release. I will show you how to go slowly and "listen" to the muscles in your body, to help you become keenly aware of the relationship between your body and mind. This will energize you. As one of my clients said,

"I'm often exhausted when I start my workout, but by the time I'm finished, my energy is booming."

Taking the Work out of Workout

Unlike many programs, I do not push you or have you set lofty goals. Instead, go at your own pace. It is better to do some exercise on a consistent basis as opposed to exercising sporadically or not at all. This program is geared toward your individual needs; it does not have arbitrary goals or standards that everyone is expected to follow. One of its main goals is to give you a sense of accomplishment from your level of achievement, which is a wonderful feeling.

In addition, as I mentioned in Chapter 2, you'll experience an improved body image, a sense of control of your life and your health, more restful sleep, time away from destructive thoughts, and a greater likelihood that you will stop addictive behaviors such as smoking and overeating.

Aerobic Exercise for Functional Fitness

While my main focus in this book is gentle strength training, I would suggest doing some form of aerobic exercise as well. Aerobic exercise is defined as anything that requires oxygen to move the large muscle groups of the body. Some examples include: indoor and outdoor biking, rowing, walking, jogging, and swimming.

Aerobic exercise gets your heart in better shape. This will help when you are playing with your children, running for the bus, or washing your car. This is called functional fitness. Being functionally fit keeps your heart and lungs healthy, while making everyday tasks easier. Being in better aerobic condition is also important for lowering stress. Haven't you heard the saying, "walk it off," after an upsetting moment?

The physical benefits of gentle strength training combined with a little aerobic exercise include: improved strength, balance and flexibility, stronger bones, a toned physique, a faster metabolism that can lead to weight loss, improved heart and lung function, positive changes in blood cholesterol, lower blood pressure, and an easing of low back pain.

While aerobic exercise is important, I certainly don't want to overwhelm you with the notion of it. You can start off with 5 minutes and work up to 25 or 30 minutes a day. If you like, divide that time into two parts with 15 minutes here and 15 minutes there.

When it comes to aerobic exercise, you know that you are exercising at the right level if you can carry on a conversation while doing it. If you are too breathless to talk, then you are exercising too hard. On the other hand, if you can sing during aerobic exercise, the intensity is not hard enough.

You can make exercise a natural part of your day by doing some of your errands on foot, or parking at the far end of the lot and walking the extra distance to the store. Or how about mowing the lawn instead of hiring a landscaper? Just make sure that you're dressed appropriately with comfortable clothes and a good pair of walking shoes. You may even want to carry a water bottle along.

For your convenience, I have also outlined walking programs in Chapters 7 through 9 that will help you progress easily and safely.

Strength-Training Lingo

Next, I'd like to familiarize you with some basic terms that I'll be using when we move to the exercise section of the book.

+ Repetition (reps): This is one, single, complete movement of the exercise. The goal is to start the movement, complete it, and return to the position that you started from. Proper execution of each movement is important to engage the specific muscle groups, and thus attain the benefit of the exercise. Good form during each repetition is essential to ensure safety and continued progress.
+ Set: This is a sequence of one or more repetitions, done consecutively. For example, when you pick up a dumbbell and curl it ten times and then put it down, that is one set of ten reps.
+ Positive movement: This is the moment of exertion during the lift, working against gravity, when the muscle contracts and shortens.
+ Peak contraction: This is the point at which the muscle is tight or contracted at the top of the movement.
+ Negative movement: This is done as the muscle lengthens, working with gravity. The idea is to control the movement, rather then letting momentum take over.

+ Isolated movement: This is an exercise that targets a single muscle group.
+ Compound movement: This is an exercise that targets one or more muscles or muscle groups.

Getting the Best Workout

While the exercises I prescribe here are on the mild side, make sure you discuss them with your physician. He or she knows your medical history and can tell you how to modify your activity, if necessary.

You'll also want to follow these important tips to ensure that you not only enjoy the exercises but that you get the maximum benefit from your efforts. It might make sense to review these suggestions now and then to make sure that you are building good exercise habits.

+ Set up a comfortable place to exercise. Make sure there is ample lighting and open a window or switch on a fan, if needed.
+ Wear comfortable clothes. Any type of loose fitting clothes is fine, along with a comfortable pair of sneakers. Fancy workout clothes are not necessary, unless putting them on makes you feel more like exercising. It depends on your personal style.
+ Turn on the music. If you prefer to exercise to your favorite CD, doing so can be motivating. Listening to the radio is also fine. I don't recommend listening to the ball game or radio talk shows, however, as they

may distract you. The key is to stay completely focused on what you are doing.

+ Warm up before you begin. Five minutes of walking or riding an exercise bike should do it.

+ Drink your water. It makes sense to keep a water bottle nearby to keep your body properly hydrated. Not only is dehydration unhealthy, it can also make you feel sluggish, and give you a headache.

+ Keep the weight light. Better to build up slowly, rather than use weights or exercise bands that are too heavy. If the weight is too heavy, your form will get sloppy and you will be more prone to injury. Don't let your ego get in the way.

+ Go easy at first. Don't set impossible goals or expect too much too fast. Start gradually. Your workout schedule should be three times a week on non-consecutive days for 30 to 45 minutes.

+ When exercising one side of your body, start with the weaker side. This is because you want to keep the number of repetitions the same. That means, if you are right handed, begin with your left side. For example, let's take the leg extension (with ankle weights). If you can only perform eight repetitions with your left leg, do only eight with your right leg, even if you feel you can do more. In this program, I will start single-side exercises, such as the leg extension, with your left side.

+ Work the larger muscle groups first, and then proceed to the smaller ones. Start with the quadriceps (front of thighs), then hamstrings (back of thighs), chest, back, shoulders, triceps (back of arms), and finish with biceps (front of upper arms).

✤ Move slowly and smoothly. Perform each repetition in a slow and deliberate manner, taking three seconds to complete the movement. At the top of the movement, when the muscle is clinched tight, hold it for two seconds. Then take four seconds, resisting gravity, as you finish the movement.

✤ Concentrate. Completely focus on the movement of each muscle during each and every repetition. Doing this allows your mind and body to fall into partnership. Before long you'll be in a zone where your mind and muscles move in harmony and gain strength together. Concentrate on how the working muscle shortens on the uptake of the weight, tightens at the top of the movement, and how it lengthens as you slowly allow gravity to pull the weight back down again.

✤ Breathe correctly through each stage of the exercise. Make sure that you breathe from your diaphragm, exhaling through your mouth as you lift the weight, and inhaling through your nose as you lower the weight. Slow, rhythmic breathing is relaxing. If done properly, it also creates the correct tension and resistance for each muscle contraction.

When you are exhaling through your mouth, imagine that you are blowing out your stress. Think of letting the tension go right out of your mouth. Once again, put your mind on the working muscle as you breathe.

Think of the muscle, every fiber of it, lengthening and tightening during the movement of the exercise. Remember, when the muscle is contracted and taut, hold the position for two seconds and feel how tight the muscle is. Exhale during the positive or lifting phase, and inhale during the negative or lowering phase.

+ Feel the rhythm. If you are consistent with these exercises, in time, you will establish a rhythm and harmony between your thoughts and your muscles. I've always felt that if you listen carefully enough, you can almost hear music being created between your mind and your body. I think of it as "breakthrough" music, great rhythms of health and understanding. This book is your sheet music. Now it's up to you to make your body sing through these exercises.

+ Progress gradually. You want to complete 8–12 repetitions for each exercise. If you have difficulty completing eight repetitions of an exercise with very strict form, it means the weight, or resistance for exercise bands, is too heavy. You are better off using a lighter weight or less resistant exercise band. If you can easily complete more than 12 repetitions, you need to increase the weight slightly—ideally, between 5 and 10 percent. In other words, if you are using a 2-pound weight, try a 2.5-pound weight.

We are aiming for a gradual progression in the build-up of your strength. Try to increase the amount of repetitions and weight (or resistance) with every workout, if possible. For example, you are doing an exercise using 2-pound weights for eight repetitions. For the next workout, you would use 2 pounds for nine repetitions. The next workout would be 2 pounds for ten repetitions, and so on. When you reach 12 reps, increase from 2 pounds to 2.5 or 3 pounds, and start with eight repetitions. In time, increase the number of sets that you complete.

The main thing is to use proper form and complete each exercise slowly.

+ Rest between sets. Take between 60 and 90 seconds. During this time, change weights if needed and get the next exercise ready to go. Remember to drink your water.

+ Stay with it. To obtain the full benefits of this program, you'll need to be consistent. The fact that you are using self-discipline will give you a sense of control over your life. If you ease into the program, with reasonable goals, you will stay with it.

+ Progress slowly and surely. It's time to abandon the all-or-nothing mentality, which will lead to injury and discouragement. Moderation is the key. Doing more is not necessarily better. I've said this many times. It's so important that I can't say it often enough.

+ Respect your body by following other healthy habits. Make sure that you eat properly and get enough sleep. You don't want poor habits in other areas of your life to cancel out the benefits of exercise. Be sure to take good care of your whole self.

You will find the actual exercises in the next four chapters. Chapter 6 will give you stretches for your whole body to make sure that you are fully warmed up. The exercises in Chapter 7 and 8 are designed for beginners and intermediates, respectively. They call for using your own body weight as well as exercise bands. Chapter 7 will be a good starting point for most readers. Chapter 9 has a more advanced routine that calls for using dumbbells.

Each of these chapters includes a month-long strength-training program to follow as well as a walking or jogging program.

Now, turn the page, and let's get started.

6

Stretching Exercises

It is a matter first of beginning—then following through.

ℊ Richard L. Evans

As you begin your stretches, keep in mind there is an art to doing this the right way.

Looking back, it was the fact that I learned to exercise in a safe, controlled, focused, and mindful manner, always using the proper form, that helped me transform my life.

It is very important to relax during the stretching routine. It should not be rushed. The I've-got-to-hurry-up attitude is counterproductive. This is a time to slow your breathing and free your mind.

Stretching is wonderful and tremendously relaxing. It helps keep your body flexible and increases your mobility, which makes the tasks of daily life easier to do. Greater flexibility can also protect you from injury, whether you are young, middle-aged, or older.

Do this program whenever you need to relax. If you're feeling stressed at work, for example, the focus that these exercises require can help to relieve your anxiety. You will want to use these exercises to loosen up your muscles before the beginning, intermediate, and advanced programs described in the next three chapters and to warm up before walking or jogging.

You can also use these stretches as a tool to get you started on days when you don't feel like exercising. Tell yourself that you're going to start with one, three, five, or all of the stretching exercises in this chapter, whatever you can handle. Chances are, if you get started, you'll get into a rhythm, and continue.

for the front of your thighs

Standing Quadricep Stretch

Position

+ Stand a few inches away from a wall or the back of a chair.
+ Place your feet hip-width apart and place your right hand against the wall or chair for support.
+ Raise your left foot behind your buttocks until you can grasp your ankle with your left hand.

Movement

+ Gently pull your heel in toward your buttocks until you feel a slight stretch in your left quadricep.
+ Move your hips slowly forward until you have reached the farthest comfortable position.

✤ Think of peaceful thoughts as you feel the muscles in
   your upper thigh lengthen.
✤ Hold for 15 seconds.
✤ Slowly return to the starting position.
✤ Repeat with your right leg.

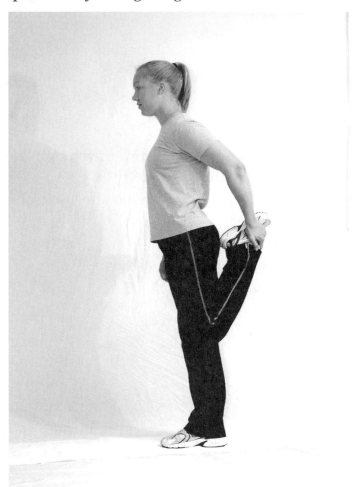

Figure 1: Standing Quadricep Stretch

for the back of your thighs

Standing Hamstring Stretch

Position

+ Stand with your feet hip-width apart in front of a table or chair.
+ Place your left heel on the table or chair so that your leg is extended straight in front of you.
+ Bend your right knee slightly.

Movement

+ Slowly lower your upper body toward your left knee to the farthest comfortable position.
+ Feel the tranquility as you stretch the back of your thigh.
+ Hold for 15 seconds.
+ Slowly return to the starting position.
+ Repeat with your right leg.

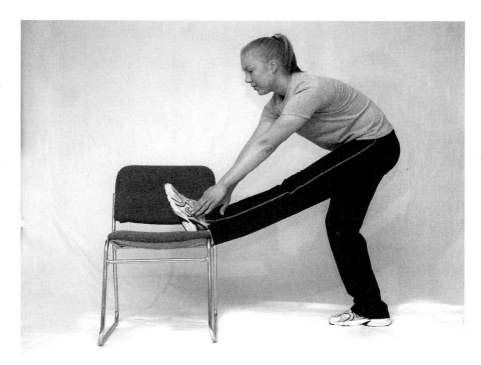

Figure 2. Standing Hamstring Stretch

for the back of your lower legs

Standing Calf Stretch

Position

+ Stand a few inches away from a wall.
+ Place your feet hip-width apart and your hands in front of you against the wall for balance.
+ Keep your back straight.
+ Step back with your left leg.
+ Bend your right leg slightly.

Movement

+ Push your left heel into the floor until you feel a pull in your calf muscle.
+ Feel a calm as your lower leg is stretching.
+ Hold for 15 seconds.
+ Repeat with your right leg.

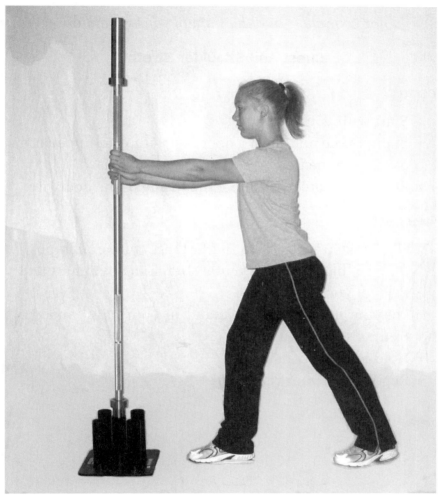

Figure 3. Standing Calf Stretch

for your chest and the front of your shoulders

Chest and Shoulder Stretch

Position

- ✦ Start with your left side.
- ✦ Stand in the middle of a doorway with your upper arm parallel to the floor.
- ✦ Place your forearm against the inside of the doorway.

Movement

- ✦ Slowly step forward to the farthest comfortable position, so that you feel a gentle stretch in your chest and front of your shoulder.
- ✦ Feel the muscle fibers expand in your chest and the front of your shoulders.
- ✦ Hold for 15 seconds.
- ✦ Repeat with your right side.

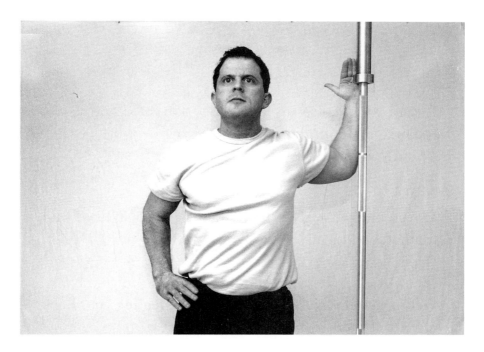

Figure 4: Chest and Shoulder Stretch

for the upper and lower back

Back Stretch

Position

+ Stand 3–4 inches from a heavy pole or other sturdy object with your feet hip-width apart.
+ Bend your knees.

Movement

+ Grasp the pole with both hands at chest level and extend your arms.
+ Lean back.
+ Look down, relax your shoulders and round your back.
+ Think serene thoughts while you are feeling your back gently stretch.
+ Hold for 15 seconds.
+ Slowly return to the starting position.

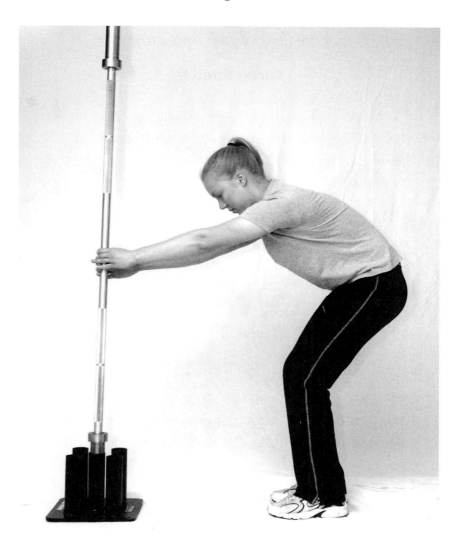

Figure 5. Back Stretch

for the back of your upper arms

Tricep Stretch

Position

- + Stand straight with your knees slightly bent.
- + Place your feet shoulder-width apart.
- + Keep your toes pointed straight ahead.
- + Keep your shoulders level.
- + Bend your left arm at your elbow joint.
- + Position your upper arm (from elbow to shoulder) next to your head with your elbow pointing out.
- + Place your left fingers on top of your shoulders or on the back of your neck.
- + Put your right hand on your left wrist.

Movement

- + Pull gently to get an added stretch.
- + Focus on the lengthening of the muscles in the back of your upper arm, think of a beautiful, peaceful place as you feel the stretch.
- + Hold for 15 seconds.
- + Slowly return to the starting position.
- + Repeat with your right arm.

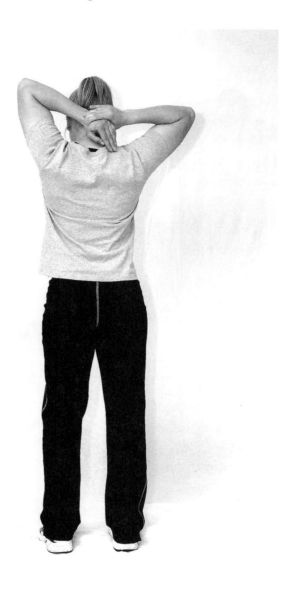

Figure 6. Tricep Stretch

for the front of your upper arms

Bicep Stretch

Position

+ Stand up straight with your knees slightly bent.
+ Place your feet hip-width apart.
+ Keep your toes pointed straight ahead.
+ Keep your shoulders level.
+ Lift your left arm to the side to shoulder level, forming a 90-degree angle between your left arm and your body.
+ Face your palm down.

Movement

+ Rotate your wrist so that your palm faces behind you and your thumb is down.
+ Concentrate on the relaxing stretch in the front of your upper arms.
+ Inhale through your nose, and exhale through your mouth.
+ Hold for 15 seconds.
+ Slowly return to the starting position.
+ Repeat with your right arm.

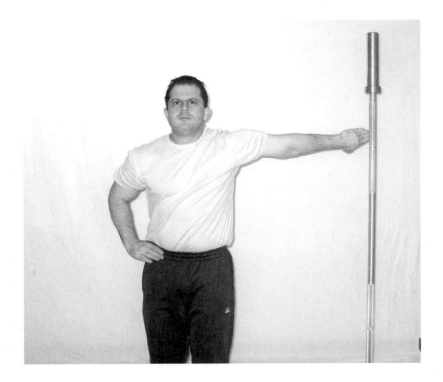

7

Beginner Program

My body must be set a-going if my mind is to work.

✌ Jean Jacques Rousseau

If you're new to exercise or haven't exercised in quite awhile, then I suggest that you start with this program. Remember exercise is not about ego—it's not about competing with yourself or others. Rather, your goal should be to start at a point where you feel comfortable and then slowly progress.

Note in the program, I recommend that you do these exercises three days a week. Rather than doing so in succession; it is much better to exercise on alternate days to give your muscles time to rest and get stronger.

I've also included a progressive, light walking program. Aerobic exercise is mentally and physically healthy, as we discuss in Chapter 5. I strongly encourage you to include walking into your exercise program, so that you can enjoy its stress-reducing benefits. You should be able to easily incorporate this into your day. Be sure to read the section in Chapter 5,"Getting the Best Workout," before you begin.

Equipment

These exercises make use of two things: your own body weight as well as rubber exercise bands that can be purchased at any department store. There are different color-coded resistance levels. Start off with the lightest resistance and gradually increase. You can also vary the resistance (increase or decrease the intensity) by shortening or lengthening the band.

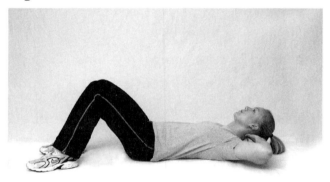

Figure 8. Crunches (A)

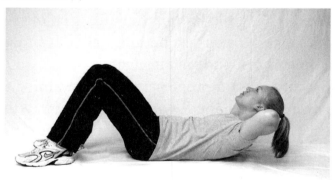

Figure 9. Crunches (B)

for your stomach

Crunches

Position

+ Lie flat on your back with your knees bent.
+ Keep your feet flat on the floor, shoulder width apart and about 10-15 inches from your buttocks.
+ Place your hands behind your ears.
+ Keep your elbows wide and your neck relaxed.
+ Keep your chin pointed to the ceiling.

Movement

+ Exhale through your mouth as you take 3 seconds to lift your shoulder blades 3 to 4 inches off the floor (if you lift higher, the focus will shift from your stomach to your lower back and hips).
+ As you lift, think of pressing your belly button into the floor and keep your lower back flat.
+ Pause for 2 seconds at the top and feel the tightening in your stomach.
+ Inhale through your nose as you slowly lower your shoulder blades towards the floor for 4 seconds without letting your hands hit the floor.

Extra Stretch: At the end of the exercise, straighten your arms and legs and think of your body lengthening. Hold for 15 seconds.

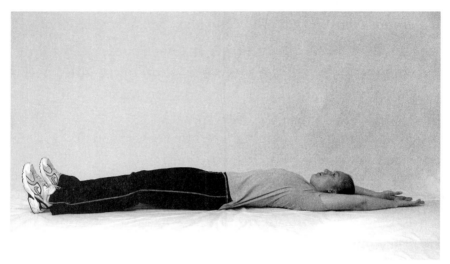

Figure 10. Crunches (Extra Stretch)

Chair Squats

This exercise concentrates on the front of your thighs. Because this is a compound movement, other muscle groups come into play, such as the back of your thighs and your buttocks.

Position

+ Place the back of one chair in front of you and the front of another chair behind you. The chair in front is for balance and the chair in back is to keep you from squatting too low.
+ Stand with feet shoulder-width apart and hands gently on the chair in front.
+ Keep your upper back straight, your head up, and look forward. This will help keep your lower back from rounding.

Movement

+ Inhale through your nose as you bend your knees, keeping your shins perpendicular to the floor; lower your butt to the chair for 4 seconds, and feel the stretch in the front of your thighs.
+ Pause for ½ second.
+ Exhale taking 3 seconds as you straighten your legs.
+ Return to the starting position with your head up, eyes forward

Extra stretch: Bend your knees, round your back, keep your head down, and feel the stretch in your lower back and the back of your thighs. Hold for 15 seconds.

Caution

＊ *If you feel any pain in your lower back or knees, stop immediately.*

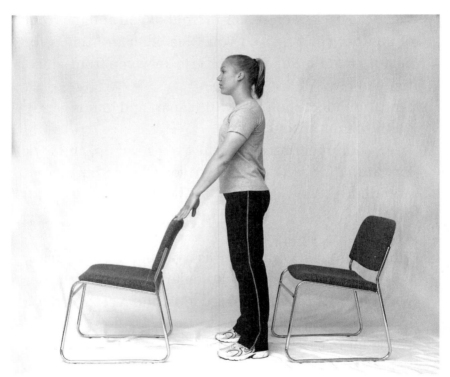

Figure 11. Chair Squats (A)

Hints

+ Do not move your knees farther forward than your toes.
+ Do not squat down so low that your thighs are below parallel to the floor.
+ Do not bounce your body in an attempt to gain momentum.
+ Do not lock your knees at the top.

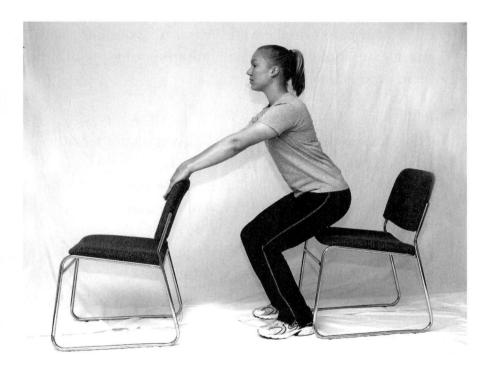

Figure 12. Chair Squats (B)

for your chest

Wall Push-Up

Position

+ Stand facing a wall with your feet hip-width apart and your knees slightly bent.
+ Keep your back straight and your stomach tight.
+ The closer your feet are to the wall, the easier the push-up movement will be.
+ Place your palms on the wall, fingers up, your hands at chest level, about 4 inches wider than shoulder-width.
+ Bend your elbows.

Movement

+ Take 3 seconds to exhale through your mouth while pushing yourself away from the wall.
+ When straightening your arms, make sure that your elbows are not locked at the top of the movement.
+ Feel the tension leaving your body.
+ Pause for ½ second.
+ Inhale through your nose, as you bend your elbows and move your body for 4 seconds until your chest touches the wall.

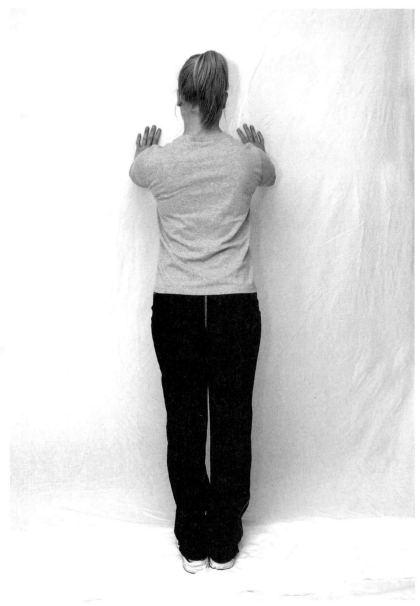

Figure 13. Wall Push-Up (A)

Extra stretch: Chest and Shoulder Stretch. Stand in the middle of a doorway with your upper arm parallel to the floor, and place your forearm against the inside of the doorway. Slowly step forward to the farthest comfortable position, so that you feel a gentle stretch in your chest and front of your shoulder.

Hold for 15 seconds. Repeat with other arm.

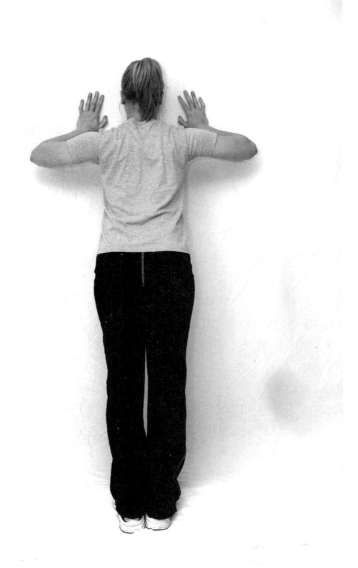

Figure 14. Wall Push-Up (B)

for the lower back

Back Extension

Position

- ✦ Lie face down on the floor.
- ✦ Keep your hands at your sides, your palms facing up, and your feet on the floor.

Movement

- ✦ Take 3 seconds as you exhale through your mouth while slowly raising your head and shoulders from the floor to a comfortable position,
- ✦ Focus on great thoughts.
- ✦ Pause for 2 seconds and feel your lower back slightly tighten as it is getting stronger.
- ✦ Inhale through your nose, as you lower your head and shoulders for 4 seconds until your chest touches the floor.

Extra stretch: Back Stretch. Stand 3 to 4 inches from a heavy pole or other sturdy object with your feet hip-width apart and knees bent. Grasp the pole with both hands at your chest level and extend your arms.

- ✦ Lean back. Look down, relax your shoulders, and round your back.
- ✦ Hold for 15 seconds.
- ✦ Slowly return to the starting position.

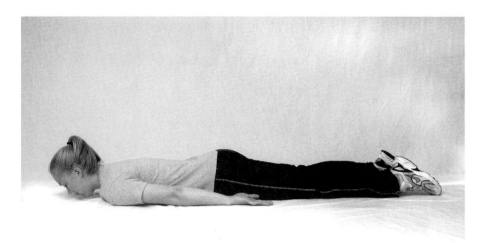

Figure 15. Back Extension (A)

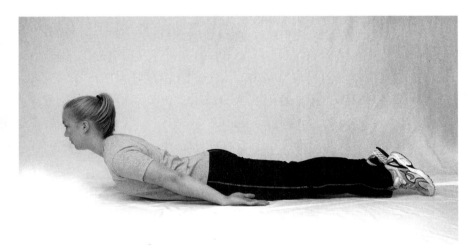

Figure 16. Back Extension (B)

for the front of your shoulders

Band Front Raise

Position

- ✤ Stand with your feet hip-width apart and your knees slightly bent.
- ✤ Keep your shoulders back, chest out, and back straight with a slight forward lean.
- ✤ Put one end of the band underneath your left foot.
- ✤ Hold the other end of the band in your left hand.
- ✤ Place right hand on hip for balance.

Movement

- ✤ Exhale through your mouth as you take 3 seconds to lift the band forward in front of your body until it is at your shoulder level, your palms facing the floor.
- ✤ Keep your wrist and elbow in line with your shoulders at the top of the movement.
- ✤ Pause for 2 seconds and feel the front of your shoulder tightening.
- ✤ Inhale through your nose as you lower the band three-quarters of the way down for 4 seconds; don't let the band touch your body as you will lose tension.

Extra stretch: Hold the band at the bottom and round your shoulders for 15 seconds, thinking of the exercise band as an anchor while you feel the stretch in your shoulders.

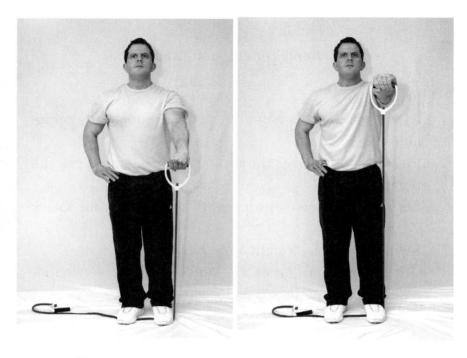

Figure 17. Band Front Raise (A)   *Figure 18. Band Front Raise (B)*

for the sides of your upper arms

Band Tricep Push-Down

Position

- Tie one end of the band to the doorknob on the opposite side of a door.
- Place the band over the top of the door and close the door.
- Stand with your feet hip-width apart and your knees slightly bent.
- Keep your back straight and your stomach tight.
- Grasp the other end of the band with your left hand, palm down, and face the closed door.
- Bend your elbow so that your forearm is parallel with the floor.
- Keep your upper arm (from elbow to shoulder) at your side throughout the movement and your wrist firm.
- Place your right hand on your hip for balance.

Movement

- Take 3 seconds exhaling through your mouth as you push downward with your left arm as far as you can without locking your elbow.
- Hold for 2 seconds in this position, feeling the side of your upper arm tightening.
- Inhale through your nose, as you raise your forearm until it is parallel to the floor (your arm at an L shape) for 4 seconds.

Extra stretch: Stop at the L shape, then raise your forearms to your chest and feel a great stretch.

Hold for 15 seconds.

Repeat with your right arm.

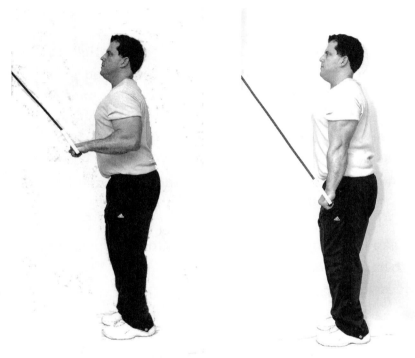

Figure 19. Band Tricep Push-Down (A)   *Figure 20. Band Tricep Push-Down (B)*

for the front of your upper arms

Band Bicep Curls

Position

+ Stand with your feet hip-width apart and your knees slightly bent.
+ Keep your back straight and your stomach tight.
+ Put one end of the band underneath your left foot.
+ Hold the other end of the band in your left hand.
+ Place your right hand on your hip for balance.
+ Use an underhand grip.
+ Keep your upper arm (from elbow to shoulder) at your side throughout the movement and your wrist firm.

Movement

+ Take 3 seconds as you pull the band up toward your chest.
+ Exhale away your troubles.
+ Keep your elbow fixed at your side, just moving your forearms.
+ At the top, your knuckles should be facing the ceiling.
+ Hold for 2 seconds and feel the front of your upper arm tightening.
+ Inhale through your nose as you slowly lower the band for 4 seconds to the starting position.

Extra stretch: To get an extra stretch, turn your wrist back slightly, and hold for 15 seconds. Repeat with your right arm.

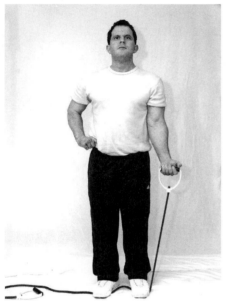

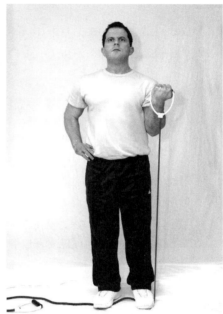

Figure 21. Band Bicep Curls (A)   *Figure 22. Band Bicep Curls (B)*

Four-Week Beginner Program

Remember:

1 x 8–12 means 1 set of 8–12 repetitions.
2 x 8–12 means 2 sets of 8–12 repetitions.

Week 1

Schedule: 3 days per week, on alternate days

+ Crunches 1 x 8–12
+ Chair Squats 1 x 8–12
+ Wall Push-Up 1 x 8–12
+ Band Tricep Push-Down 1 x 8–12
+ Band Bicep Curls 1 x 8–12

Walk 5 minutes (3 days per week)

Week 2

Schedule: 3 days per week, on alternate days

+ Crunches 1 x 8–12
+ Chair Squats 1 x 8–12
+ Wall Push-Up 2 x 8–12
+ Back Extension 1 x 8–12
+ Band Tricep Push-Down 1 x 8–12
+ Band Bicep Curls 1 x 8–12

Walk 8 minutes (3 days per week)

Week 3

Schedule: 3 days per week, on alternate days

+ Crunches 2 x 8–12
+ Chair Squats 2 x 8–12
+ Wall Push-Up 2 x 8–12
+ Back Extension 2 x 8–12
+ Band Front Raise 1 x 8–12
+ Band Tricep Push-Down 2 x 8–12
+ Band Bicep Curls 1 x 8–12

Walk 10 minutes (3 days a week)

Week 4

Schedule: 3 days per week, on alternate days

+ Crunches 2 x 8–12
+ Chair Squats 2 x 8–12
+ Wall Push-Up 2 x 8–12
+ Back Extension 2 x 8–12
+ Band Front Raise 2 x 8–12
+ Band Tricep Push-Down 2 x 8–12
+ Band Bicep Curls 2 x 8–12

Walk 12 minutes (3 days a week)

8

Intermediate Program

Our greatest glory is not in failing, but in rising every time we fail.

ॐ Confucius

If you have experience with exercise or have completed the beginner program, it is time to try the intermediate program. Remember, go at your own pace.

You will learn new exercises in this chapter with added sets. You will also increase your time walking and start your jogging routine. Review the section in Chapter 5 on Getting the Best Workout before you start.

Equipment

These exercises will require the same equipment used in the beginner program: your own body weight and rubber exercise bands.

for your lower stomach

Crunches with Feet Raised

Position

- ✦ Lie on your back.
- ✦ Raise your lower legs off the ground or place your feet on a chair or table to make the exercise less difficult.
- ✦ Make sure that your thighs are perpendicular to the floor.
- ✦ Place your hands behind your ears.
- ✦ Keep your elbows wide and your neck relaxed.
- ✦ Keep your chin pointed to the ceiling.

Movement

- ✦ Exhale through your mouth as you slowly raise your shoulder blades 3-4 inches off the ground (if you lift higher, the focus will shift from your stomach to your lower back and hips).
- ✦ As you are lifting, think of pressing your belly button into the floor and keep your lower back flat.
- ✦ Pause for 2 seconds and feel the tightening in your stomach.
- ✦ Inhale through your nose, taking 4 seconds to slowly lower your shoulder blades without letting your hands hit the floor.

Extra stretch: Straighten your arms and legs and think of your body lengthening. Hold for 15 seconds.

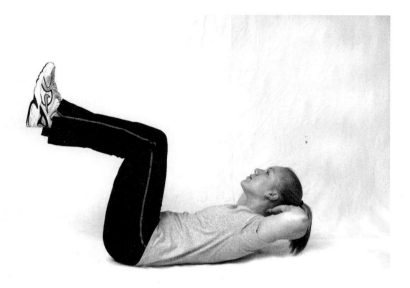

Figure 23. Crunches with Feet Raised

Bodyweight Squats

This exercise concentrates on the front of your thighs. Because this is a compound movement, other muscle groups come into play, such as the backs of your thighs and your buttocks.

Position

+ Stand upright with your arms in front of your body for balance.
+ Stand with your feet about hip-width apart.
+ Keep your upper back straight, your head up, and look forward. (This will help keep your lower back from rounding.)

Movement

+ Inhale as you bend your knees, keeping your shins per-pendicular to the floor; lower your butt for 4 seconds until your thighs are almost parallel to the floor.
+ Feel the stretch in the front of your thighs.
+ Pause for ½ second.
+ Return to the starting position.
+ Exhale as you straighten your legs, taking 3 seconds to complete the exhale.

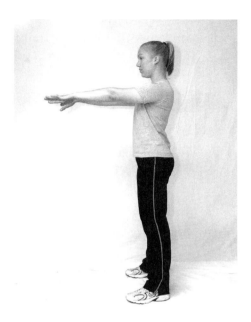

Figure 24. Bodyweight Squats (A)

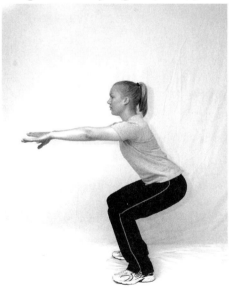

Figure 25. Bodyweight Squats (B)

Extra stretch: Bend your knees, round your back, keep your head down, and feel the stretch in your lower back and the back of your thighs.

Hold for 15 seconds.

Hints

+ Do not allow your knees to go farther forward than your toes.
+ Do not allow your thighs to go below parallel to the floor at the bottom of the movement.
+ Do not bounce your body in an attempt to gain momentum.
+ Do not lock your knees at the top.

Caution

+ If you feel any pain in your lower back or knees, stop immediately.

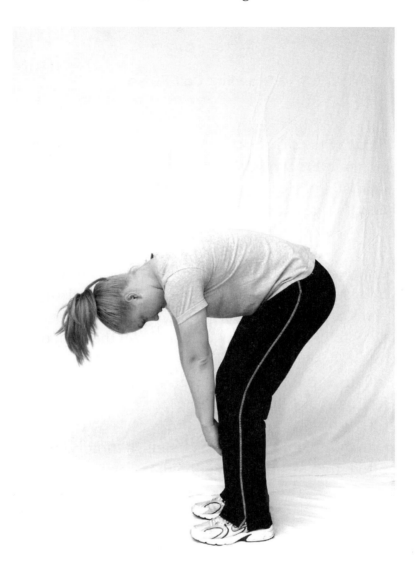

Figure 26. Rounded Back Stretch

for your calves

Standing Calf Raise

Position

+ Stand with the balls of your feet on the edge of a bottom step or other raised surface.
+ Lean slightly forward with your hands against a wall or door for balance.

Movement

+ Exhale, taking 3 seconds as you lift your body upward by extending your foot at the ankle and raising your heels as far as possible.
+ Hold for 2 seconds at the top and feel the back of your lower legs tightening.
+ Inhale as you lower your heels for 4 seconds, feeling your calves stretching.

Extra stretch: At the end of the exercise, hold your heels at the bottom for 15 seconds, feeling the stretch in your calves.

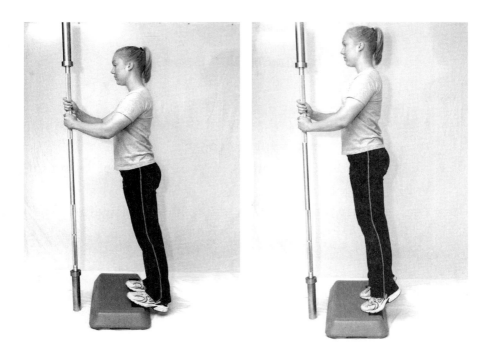

Figure 27. Standing Calf Raise (A)   *Figure 28. Standing Calf Raise (B)*

for your calves

Single-Leg Calf Raise

Position

- ✦ Stand with the ball of your left foot on the edge of a raised surface or bottom step near a door or a wall.
- ✦ Keep your right leg bent and your right foot behind you.
- ✦ Lean slightly forward, with your right hand against the wall for balance.

Movement

- ✦ Exhale as you take 3 seconds to lift your left heel upward by extending your foot at the ankle and raise your heel as far as possible.
- ✦ Hold for 2 seconds at the top and feel the back of your lower leg tightening.
- ✦ Inhale as you lower your heel for 4 seconds and feel your calf stretching.

Extra stretch: Hold your heel at the bottom for 15 seconds. Repeat with your right calf.

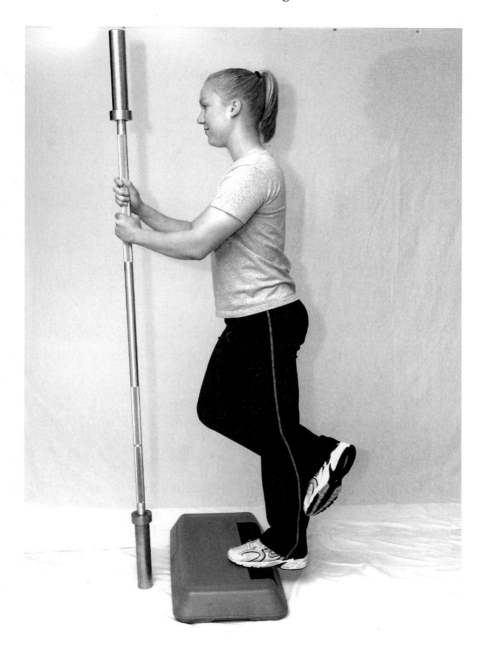

Figure 29. Single-Leg Calf Raise

for your chest

Bent-Knee Push-Up

Position

- Lie on the floor, face down.
- Place your hands at chest level about 4 inches wider than shoulder-width.
- Keep your elbows out to the side, fingers pointed straight ahead.
- Place your knees on the floor and your feet in the air.
- Keep your back straight and your stomach tight.

Movement

- Exhale, taking 3 seconds to push yourself up, straightening your arms without locking your elbows at the top.
- Pause for ½ second at the top.
- Inhale, taking 4 seconds to lower your body until your chest touches the floor.

Extra stretch: Chest and Shoulder Stretch. Stand in the middle of a doorway with your upper arm parallel to the floor, and place your forearm against the inside of the doorway. Slowly step forward to the farthest comfortable position, so that you feel a gentle stretch in your chest and front of your shoulder.

Hold for 15 seconds.

Repeat with other arm.

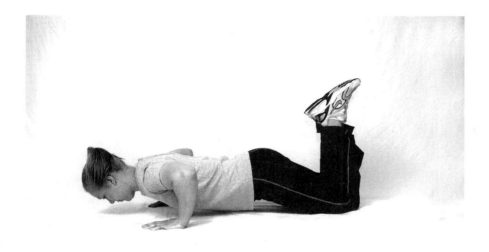

Figure 30. Bent-Knee Push Up (A)

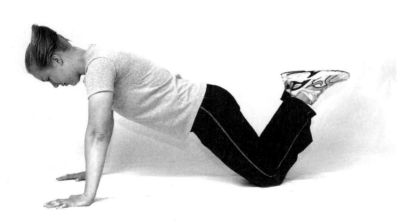

Figure 31. Bent-Knee Push Up (B)

for your chest

Standard Push-Up

Position

+ Lie on the floor, face down.
+ Place your hands at chest level about 4 inches farther than shoulder-width apart.
+ Keep your elbows out to the side, fingers pointed straight ahead.
+ Place your feet on the floor
+ Keep your back straight and stomach tight.

Movement

+ Exhale, taking 3 seconds to push yourself up, straightening your arms without locking your elbows at the top.
+ Pause for ½ second at the top.
+ Inhale, taking 4 seconds to lower your body until your chest touches the floor.

Extra stretch: Chest and Shoulder Stretch. Stand in the middle of a doorway with your upper arm parallel to the floor, and place your forearm against the inside of the doorway. Slowly step forward to the farthest comfortable position, so that you feel a gentle stretch in your chest and front of your shoulder.

Hold for 15 seconds.

Repeat with other arm.

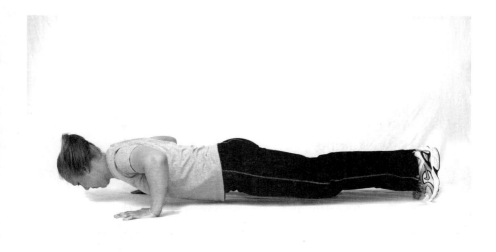

Figure 32. Standard Push-Up (A)

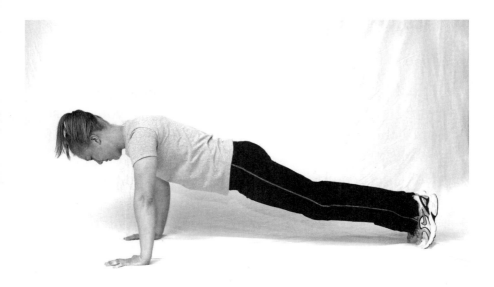

Figure 33. Standard Push-Up (B)

for your chest

Chest Crossover

Position

- ✦ Tie one end of the band to the doorknob on the opposite side of a door.
- ✦ Place the band over the top of the door and close the door.
- ✦ Grasp the handle of the exercise band with your left hand, and stand far enough away so that when your arm is extended you feel tension in the band.
- ✦ Your feet should be hip-width apart, your knees slightly bent, and your body leaning slightly forward.
- ✦ Your left hand should be at shoulder-level with your elbow slightly bent and your palm facing down.

Movement

- ✦ Exhale, taking 3 seconds as you pull the band downward in an arc, squeezing the left side of your chest until the handle is directly in front of the middle of your chest.
- ✦ Hold this position for 2 seconds; feel a slight tightening on the left side of your chest.
- ✦ Inhale as you raise your arm up to your shoulder.

Extra stretch: Step forward, raise your arm to your ear, keep your shoulders level, and feel the stretch in your chest. Hold for 15 seconds.

Repeat with your right arm.

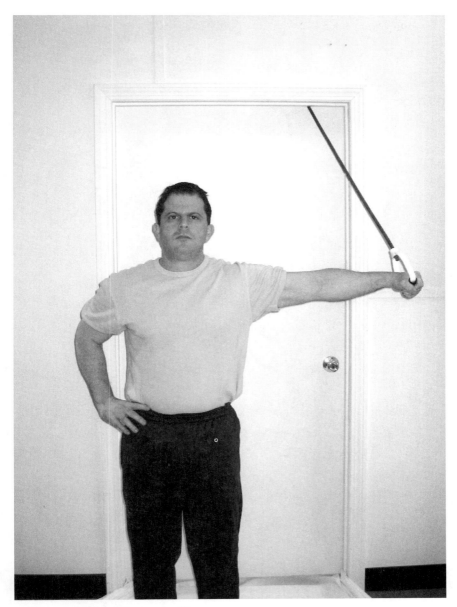

Figure 34. Chest Crossover (A)

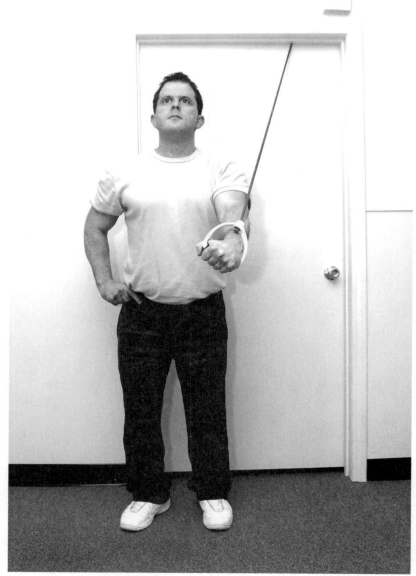

Figure 35. Chest Crossover (B)

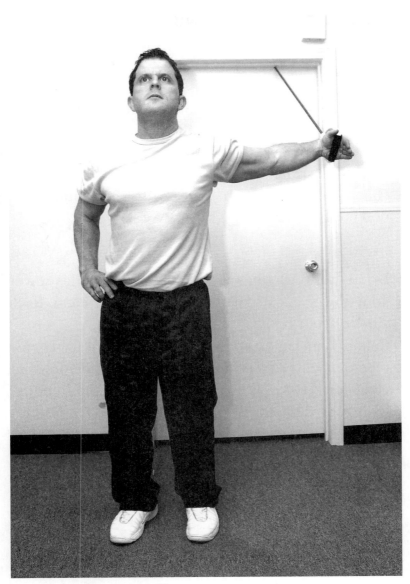

Figure 36. Chest Crossover ©)

for the middle of your back

Band Seated Row

Position

- ✤ Place the band around a heavy pole or other sturdy object about 6 inches from the floor.
- ✤ Sit with your heels on the floor, your knees bent, and your back straight.
- ✤ Grasp each handle of the band with your palms facing down.

Movement

- ✤ Exhale for 3 seconds as you pull the handles toward your lower chest, keeping your elbows close to the sides of your body.
- ✤ Rotate your hands so that your palms are facing each other, imagine squeezing your shoulder blades together.
- ✤ Hold for 2 seconds at the top and feel the middle of your back tightening.
- ✤ Inhale, taking 4 seconds to return to the starting position without letting the band pull you forward.

Extra stretch: Lean forward and round your back. Hold for 15 seconds.

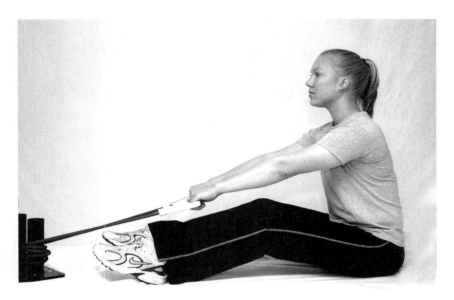

Figure 37. Band Seated Row (A)

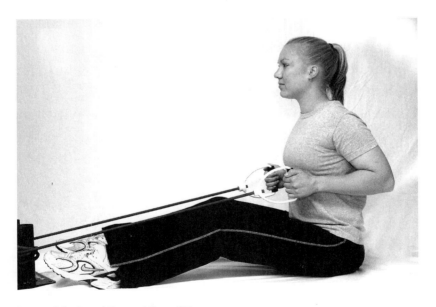

Figure 38. Band Seated Row (B)

for the sides of your shoulders

Band Side Raise

Position

+ Stand with your feet hip-width apart and your knees slightly bent.
+ Keep your shoulders back, chest out, and back straight with a slight forward lean.
+ Place one end of an exercise band underneath your left foot.
+ Hold the other end of the exercise band in your left hand.
+ Place your right hand on your hip for balance.

Movement

+ Exhale, taking 3 seconds to raise the band to the side of your body until it is at your shoulder level, your palm facing the floor.
+ Be sure to keep your wrist and elbow in line with your shoulder at the top of the movement.
+ Pause for 2 seconds and feel the tightening in the middle of your shoulder.
+ Inhale, taking 4 seconds as you lower the band in toward your body.
+ Come down only three-quarters of the way.

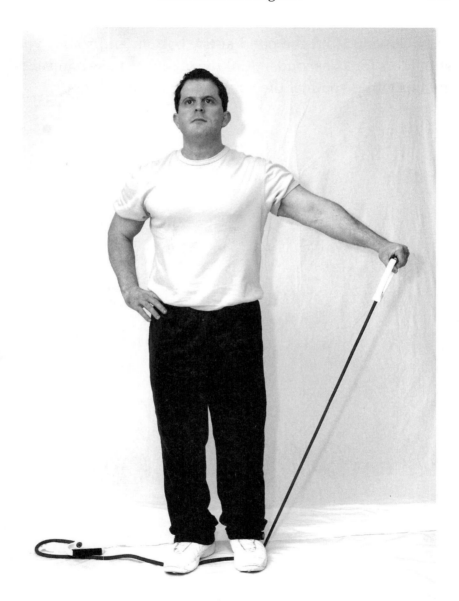

Figure 39. Band Side Raise (A)

Extra stretch: Hold the band at the bottom and round your shoulders for 15 seconds, thinking of the exercise band as an anchor while you feel the stretch in your shoulders.

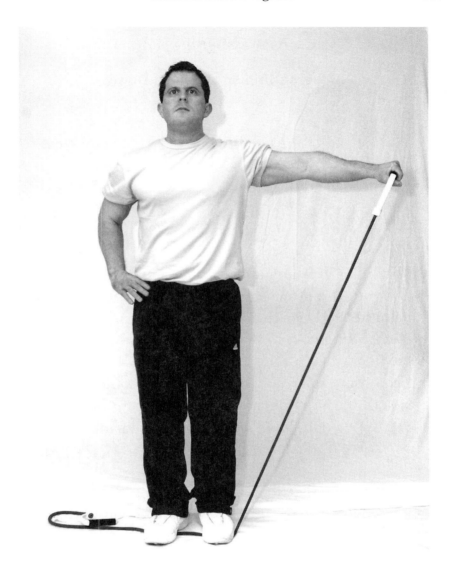

Figure 40. Band Side Raise (B)

for the back of your upper arms

Reverse-Grip Tricep Push-Down

Position

+ Tie one end of the band to the doorknob on the opposite side of a door.
+ Place the band over the top of the door and close the door.
+ Stand your feet hip-width apart and your knees slightly bent.
+ Keep your back straight and your stomach tight.
+ Grasp the other end of the band with your left hand, palm up, and face the closed door.
+ Bend your elbow so that your forearm is parallel with the floor.
+ Keep your upper arm (from elbow to shoulder) at your side throughout the movement and your wrist firm.
+ Place your right hand on your hip for balance.

Movement

+ Take 3 seconds exhaling through your mouth as you push downward with your left arm as far as you can without locking your elbow.
+ Hold for 2 seconds in this position, feeling the back of your upper arm tightening.
+ Inhale through your nose as you raise your forearm until it is parallel to the floor (your arm at an L shape) for 4 seconds.

Extra stretch: Stop at the L shape, then raise your forearm to your chest and feel a great stretch.

Hold for 15 seconds.

Repeat with your right arm.

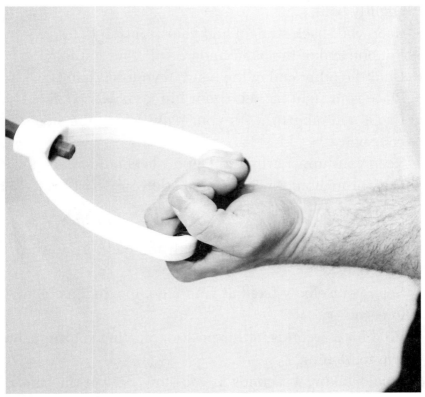

Figure 41. Reverse-Grip Tricep Push-Down

for the front of your upper arms

Band Hammer Curls

Position

- ✤ Stand with your feet hip-width apart and your knees slightly bent.
- ✤ Keep your back straight and your stomach tight.
- ✤ Put one end of the band underneath your left foot.
- ✤ Hold the other end of the band in your left hand.
- ✤ Place your right hand on your hip for balance.
- ✤ Use a neutral grip, with your palm facing the side of your body.
- ✤ Keep your upper arm (from elbow to shoulder) at your side throughout the movement and your wrist firm.

Movement

- ✤ Exhale, taking 3 seconds to pull the band up toward your chest.
- ✤ Keep your elbow fixed at your side, moving just your forearm.
- ✤ Hold for 2 seconds in this position, feeling your upper arm tightening.
- ✤ Inhale, taking 4 seconds as you slowly lower the band to the starting position in a controlled manner.

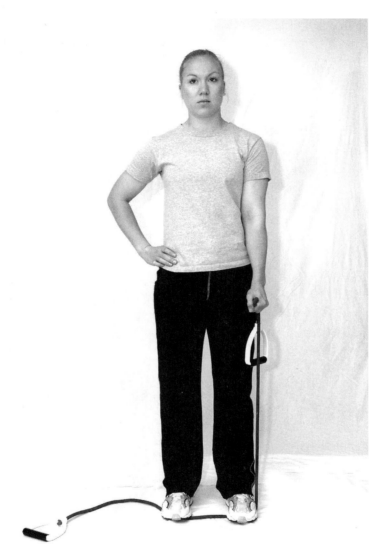

Figure 42. Band Hammer Curls (A)

Extra stretch: At the end of the movement, turn your palm forward and your wrist slightly backward and hold for 15 seconds.

Repeat with your right arm.

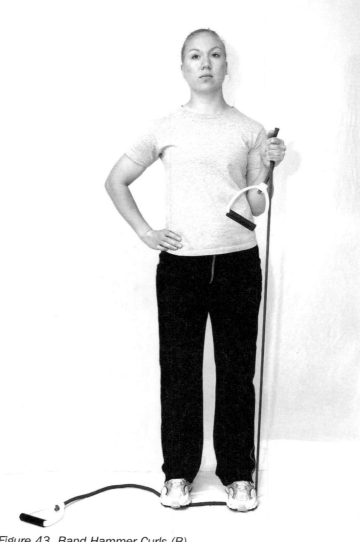

Figure 43. Band Hammer Curls (B)

Four-Week Intermediate Program

Remember:

1 x 8–12 means 1 set of 8–12 repetitions
2 x 8–12 means 2 sets of 8–12 repetitions

Week 1

Schedule: 3 days per week,
Monday, Wednesday, and Friday

+ Crunches with Feet Raised 1 x 8–12
+ Body Weight Squats 1 x 8–12
+ Standing Calf Raise 1 x 8–12
+ Bent-Knee Push-Up 1 x 8–12
+ Band Seated Row 1 x 8–12
+ Band Side Raise 1 x 8–12
+ Band Reverse Grip Tricep Push-Down 1 x 8–12
+ Band Hammer Curls 1 x 8–12

Walk 15 minutes (3 days per week),
Tuesday, Thursday, and Saturday

Week 2

Schedule: 3 days per week,
Monday, Wednesday, and Friday

- ✤ Crunches with Feet Raised 2 x 8–12
- ✤ Body Weight Squats 2 x 8–12
- ✤ Standing Calf Raise 2 x 8–12
- ✤ Bent Knee Push-Up 2 x 8–12
- ✤ Chest Crossover 1 x 8–12
- ✤ Band Seated Row 2 x 8–12
- ✤ Band Side Raise 2 x 8–12
- ✤ Band Reverse Grip Tricep Push-Down 2 x 8–12
- ✤ Band Hammer Curls 2 x 8–12

Walk 18 minutes (3 days per week)
Tuesday, Thursday, and Saturday

Week 3

Schedule: 3 days per week,
Monday, Wednesday, and Friday

+ Crunches with Feet Raised 2 x 8–12
+ Body Weight Squats 2 x 8–12
+ Single Leg Standing Calf Raise 1 x 8–12
  (Make sure that you are able to complete 2 sets of 12 repetitions with the Standing Calf Raise before trying these)
+ Standard Push-Up 1 x 8–12
  (Make sure that you are able to complete 2 sets of 12 repetitions with Bent-Knee Push-Ups before trying these)
+ Chest Crossover 1 x 8–12
+ Band Seated Row 2 x 8–12
+ Band Side Raise 2 x 8–12
+ Band Reverse Grip Tricep Push-Down 2 x 8–12
+ Band Hammer Curls 2 x 8–12

Walk 20 minutes (3 days per week)
Tuesday, Thursday, and Saturday

Week 4

Schedule: 3 days per week,
Monday, Wednesday, and Friday

- ✦ Crunches with Feet Raised 2 x 8–12
- ✦ Body Weight Squats 2 x 8–12
- ✦ Single Leg Standing Calf Raise 2 x 8–12
- ✦ Standard Push-Up 2 x 8–12
- ✦ Chest Crossover 2 x 8–12
- ✦ Band Seated Row 2 x 8–12
- ✦ Band Side Raise 2 x 8–12
- ✦ Band Reverse Grip Tricep Push-Down 2 x 8–12
- ✦ Band Hammer Curls 2 x 8–12

Alternate walking for 2 minutes with jogging for 30 seconds for a total of 20 minutes (3 days per week) Tuesday, Thursday, and Saturday.

9

Advanced Program

Physical fitness is not only the key to a healthy body; it is the basis of a dynamic and intellectual activity. Intelligence and skill can only function at the peak of their capacity when the body is strong. Hardy spirits and tough minds usually inhabit sound bodies.

    ❀ John F. Kennedy

Equipment

This program makes use of dumbbells, adjustable ankle weights, and either an adjustable step or weight bench.

If you do not already have a set of dumbbells, there are several options to choose from.

You may want to start off with just one light set of dumbbells, perhaps a one-pound set, and purchase heavier weights as you progress. You may choose to buy an adjustable pair of dumbbells that will allow you to change the weight, although this can be time-consuming.

Another option is PowerBlock®dumbbells, which are "selectorized." You just insert a pin in order to change the weight. PlateMate® makes magnetic weights that attach to the end of your dumbbells and are available from 5/8 to 5 pounds. These allow you to make a more gradual increase in the amount of weight you lift. PlateMate®and PowerBlock® products can be found in exercise equipment stores or can be purchased directly from the company.

Before You Start

Review the section in Chapter 5 on Getting the Best Workout.

for your lower stomach

Crunches with Feet Raised

Position

- ✤ Lie on your back.
- ✤ Raise your lower legs off the ground; make sure that your thighs are perpendicular to the floor.
- ✤ Place your hands behind your ears.
- ✤ Keep your elbows wide and your neck relaxed.
- ✤ Keep your chin pointed to the ceiling.

Movement

- ✤ Exhale as you slowly raise your shoulders 3–4 inches off the ground (if you lift higher, the focus will shift from your stomach to your lower back and hips).
- ✤ As you lift, think of pressing your belly button into the floor, and keep your lower back flat.
- ✤ Pause for 2 seconds and feel the tightening in your stomach.
- ✤ Inhale through your nose, taking 4 seconds to lower your shoulders without letting your hands hit the floor.

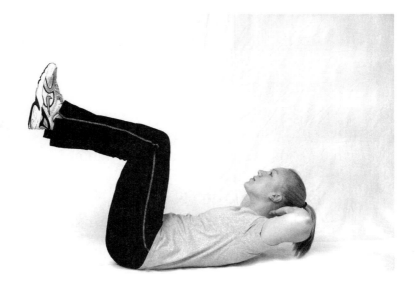

Figure 44. Crunches with Feet Raised

Extra stretch: Straighten your arms and legs and think of your body lengthening. Hold for 15 seconds.

Dumbbell Side Bend

For the sides of your waist. This exercise works the side of your waist that is opposite the hand you hold the dumbbell in.

Position

+ Stand upright while holding a light dumbbell in your right hand.
+ Place your feet about hip-width apart and your knees slightly bent.
+ Place your left hand on your waist.

Movement

+ Inhale as you bend to the side for 4 seconds, feeling the stretch on the left side of your waist.
+ Make sure that you do not lean forward.
+ Pause for 2 seconds and feel the left side of your waist stretching.
+ Exhale, taking 3 seconds to straighten your upper body.
+ Repeat holding the dumbbell in your left hand.

Extra stretch: Bend your knees, round your back, keep your head down, and feel the stretch in the lower back and side of your waist. Hold for 15 seconds.

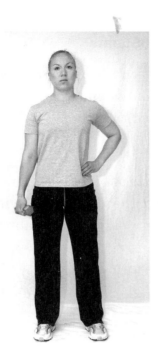
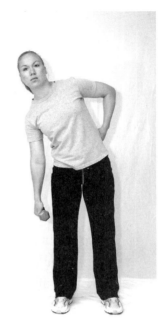

Figure 45. Dumbbell Side Bend (A)   *Figure 46. Dumbbell Side Bend (B)*

Dumbbell Squats

For the front of your thighs. Because this is a compound movement, other muscle groups come into play, such as the back of your thighs and your buttocks.

Position

+ Place the dumbbells on your shoulders. (To make the exercise less difficult hold the dumbbells with your arms extended down at your sides, your palms facing in.)
+ Place your feet about hip-width apart.
+ Keep your upper back straight, your head up, and look forward.

Movement

+ Inhale for 4 seconds as you bend your knees, keeping your shins perpendicular to the floor; lower your butt until your thighs are almost parallel to the floor; feel the stretch in the front of your thighs.
+ Pause for ½ second.
+ Exhale, taking 3 seconds as you straighten your legs.

Extra stretch: Hold the dumbbells at your side, bend your knees, round your back, keep your head down, feel the stretch in your lower back and back of your thighs. Hold for 15 seconds.

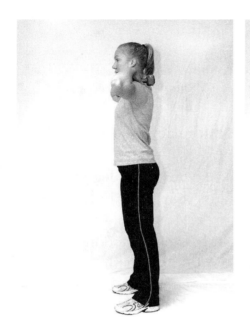 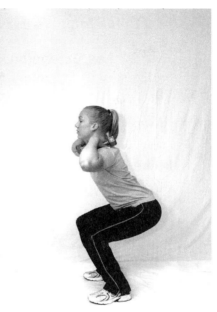

Figure 47. Dumbbell Squats (A)   *Figure 48. Dumbbell Squats (B)*

Caution

+ If you feel any pain in your lower back or knees, stop immediately.

Hints

+ Do not allow your thighs to go below parallel to the floor at the bottom of the movement.
+ Do not bounce your body in an attempt to gain momentum or lock your knees at the top.

For the front of your thighs above your knees.

Leg Extension with Ankle Weights

Position

+ Sit on a chair, pressing your butt against the back of the seat; keep your back straight.
+ Make sure you are able to drop your lower leg perpendicular to the floor without your foot hitting the ground.
+ Relax your feet, keeping your toes neutral; don't point them up (this will be tightening your shin area) or down (which will tighten your calf muscle).
+ Keep your left hand on your left thigh for balance.

Movement

+ Starting with your left thigh, exhale for three seconds while slowly straightening your lower leg (from your knee to your foot).
+ Lift all the way up without locking your knee.
+ Hold at the top for 2 seconds as you feel the muscles above your knee tightening.
+ Inhale for 4 seconds while lowering your leg; feel the stretch in the front of your thigh.
+ At the bottom of the movement, be sure your lower leg (from your knee to your foot) is perpendicular with the floor.

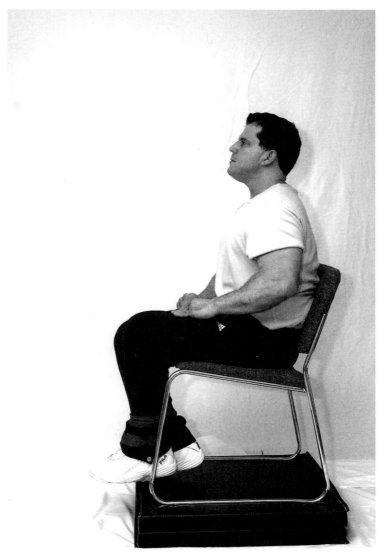

Figure 49. Leg Extension with Ankle Weights (A)

Extra stretch: In order to get an extra stretch, move your lower leg in deeper. Hold for 15 seconds. Repeat with your right leg.

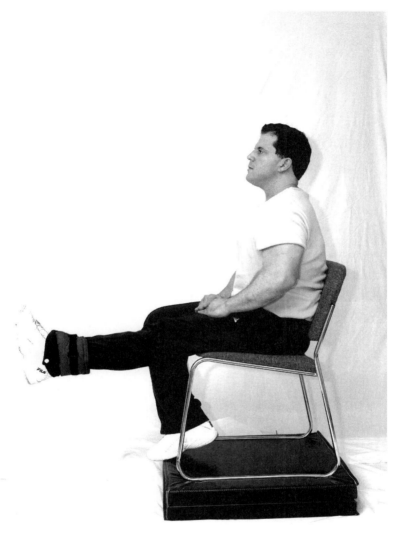

Figure 50. Leg Extension with Ankle Weights (B)

for the back of your thighs

Leg Curl with Ankle Weights

Position

+ Stand on a platform or step so you have a full range of motion during the exercise.
+ Place your right hand on the wall for support, with your feet no more than shoulder-width apart.
+ Keep your back straight.
+ Relax your feet, keeping your toes neutral; don't point them up (which will tighten your shin area) or down (which will tighten your calf muscle).
+ Keep your left hand on your left thigh to keep it from moving.

Movement

+ Exhale for 3 seconds, slowly pulling your left leg (from your knees to your feet) as close to your buttocks as you can.
+ Hold at the top for 2 seconds as you feel the back of your thighs toning.
+ Inhale for 4 seconds as you slowly lower your leg concentrating on the stretching of the back of your thigh.

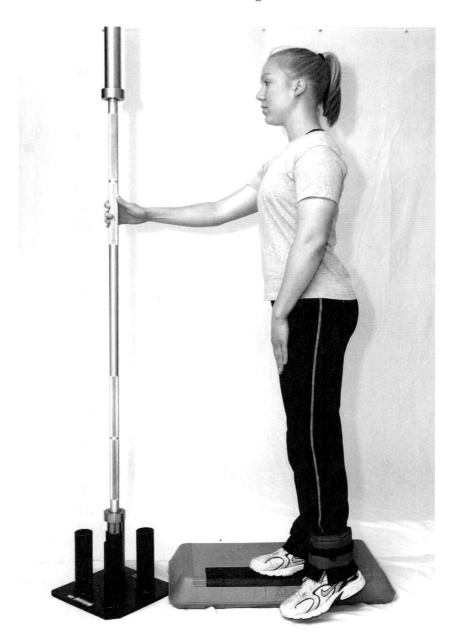

Figure 51. Leg Curl with Ankle Weights (A)

Extra stretch: Standing with your feet hip-width apart in front of a chair or table, place your left heel on the chair so that your leg is extended straight in front of you, knee bent slightly. Slowly turn lower your upper body toward your left knee to the farthest comfortable position. Feel the tranquility as you stretch the back of your thigh. Hold for 15 seconds. Repeat with your right leg.

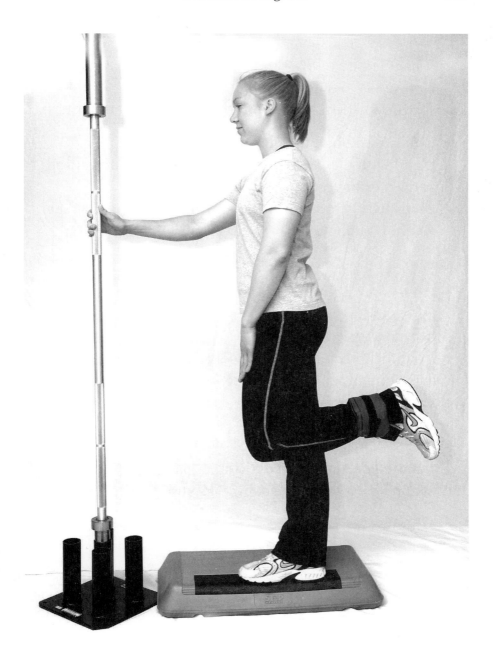

Figure 52. Leg Curl with Ankle Weights (B)

for your calves

Dumbbell Calf Raise

Position

- ✦ Hold a dumbbell in your left hand.
- ✦ Stand with the balls of your feet on the edge of a raised surface or bottom step.
- ✦ Lean slightly forward, with your right hand against the wall for balance.

Movement

- ✦ Exhale, taking 3 seconds as you lift your body upward by extending your feet at the ankle and raising your heels as far as possible.
- ✦ Hold for 2 seconds as you feel the back of your lower legs tightening.
- ✦ Inhale as you lower your heels for 4 seconds, and feel your calves stretching.

Extra stretch: At the end of the exercise, hold your heels at the bottom for 15 seconds, feeling the stretch in your calves.

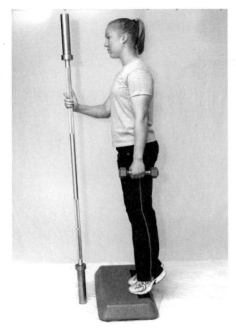 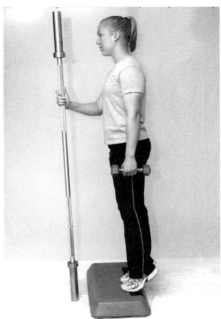

Figure 53. Dumbbell Calf Raise (A)   *Figure 54. Dumbbell Calf Raise (B)*

for the middle of your chest

Dumbbell Bench Press

Because this is a compound movement, other muscle groups come into play, such as the front of your shoulders, the back of your arms (triceps), and your forearms.

Position

+ Lie on an exercise step, or weight bench, with your legs slightly parted and your feet firmly on the floor.
+ Hold two dumbbells with your arms extended, your palms facing away from your face.
+ The dumbbells should be nearly touching each other above your chest.
+ Your back and shoulders should be straight and firm against the step, and your elbows should be unlocked.

Movement

+ Inhale while lowering the dumbbells to the sides of your chest for 4 seconds until your upper arms (from elbow to shoulder) are parallel to the floor.
+ Pause for ½ second.
+ Exhale, taking 3 seconds as you raise (push) the dumbbells up to the starting position while tightening your chest.
+ Make sure not to arch your back or bang the weights together at the top.

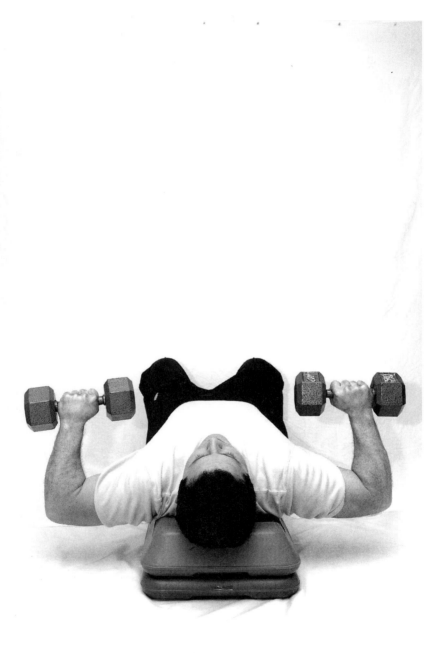

Figure 55. Dumbbell Bench Press (A)

Extra stretch: At the end of the exercise, come down very slowly and hold the weight for 15 seconds at the bottom, letting your elbows shift slightly backward.

Caution

+ Make sure you do this very slowly and controlled, and never with a jerk. Do not rotate your shoulders too far back (just enough to feel a slight stretch). Make sure your hips and shoulders are in contact with the step or bench. When finished, place the dumbbell on the floor gently.

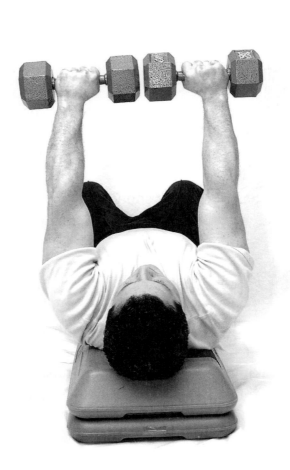

Figure 56. Dumbbell Bench Press (B)

Dumbbell Incline Bench Press

For the middle of your upper chest. Because this is a compound movement, other muscle groups come into play, such as the front of your shoulders, the back of your arms (triceps) and your forearms.

Position

+ Lie on a raised step or incline bench (about 30 degrees) with your legs slightly parted and your feet firmly on the floor.
+ Hold two dumbbells with arms extended, palms facing away from your face.
+ The dumbbells should be nearly touching each other above your chest.
+ Your back and shoulders should be firmly against the bench, and your elbows should be unlocked.

Movement

+ Inhale for 4 seconds as you lower the dumbbells to the sides of your upper chest until your upper arms (from elbow to shoulder) are parallel to the floor.
+ Pause for ½ second.
+ Exhale, taking 3 seconds as you raise (push) the weights to the starting position while tightening your chest.
+ Don't arch your back or bang the weights together at the top.

Extra stretch: Come down very slowly and hold the weight for 15 seconds at the bottom, letting your elbows shift slightly backward.

Caution

✢ At the end of the movement during the extra stretch make sure you do this very slowly and controlled, never with a quick jerk. Don't rotate your shoulders too far back (just enough to feel a slight stretch). Make sure your hips and shoulders are in contact with the step or bench.

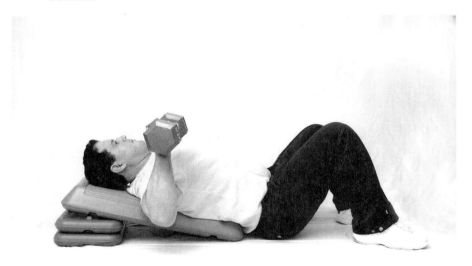

Figure 57. Dumbbell Incline Bench Press

One-Arm Dumbbell Row

This exercise concentrates on the side of your back. Since it is a compound movement other muscle groups come into play such as the back of your shoulders, the front of your arms (biceps) and your forearms.

Position

+ With your left foot firmly on the floor, hold a dumbbell in your left hand, letting your arm hang down directly in line with your shoulder joint.
+ Keep your back straight.
+ Place your right hand and your right knee on a chair for balance.
+ Look straight ahead.

Movement

+ Exhaling, take 3 seconds as you pull the weight up and in towards your body next to your lower chest.
+ Raise the weight as high as you can. Your left elbow should be pointing up toward the ceiling as you lift.
+ Think of squeezing your shoulder blades into your spine at the top of the movement.
+ Hold for 2 seconds, feeling the left side of your back tightening.
+ Inhale for 4 seconds as you lower your arm.

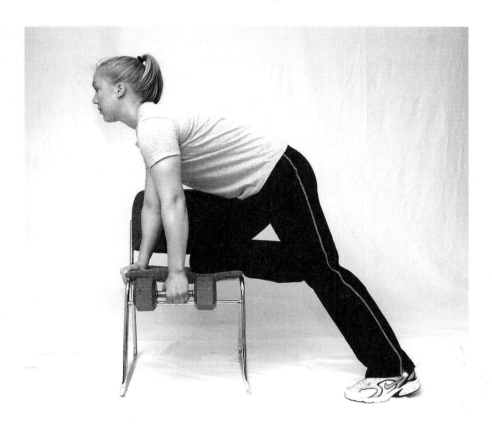

Figure 58. One-Arm Dumbbell Row (A)

Extra stretch: Hold the dumbbell (think of it as an anchor) and round your back, feeling the stretch all through your back. Hold for 15 seconds.

Repeat with your right side.

Hints

✤ Do not let the weight fall as you lower it. Lower the weight in a slow, controlled manner.

✤ Do not jerk the weight up to position. Keep it in control at all times and enjoy the sensation of your back tightening and the relief you feel when it stretches.

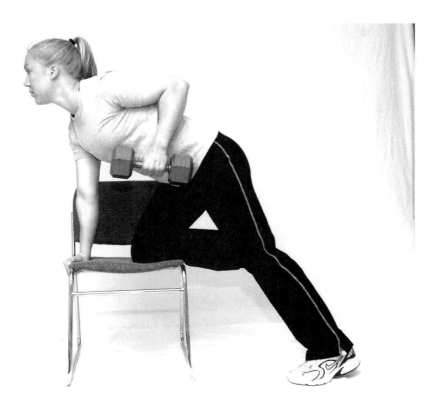

Figure 59. One-Arm Dumbbell Row (B)

for your lower back and backs of your legs (hamstrings)

Dumbbell Deadlift

Caution

+ If you have had any lower back problems, do not do this movement.

Position

+ Stand upright with a dumbbell in each hand in front of you, and your palms facing back.
+ Your feet should be about 6 inches apart, with a slight bend to them.
+ Your torso should be straight, with your lower back maintaining a natural, inward curve as you bend over at the waist.

Movement

+ Slowly bend forward until you feel a slight stretch in the back of your thighs.
+ Inhale, taking 4 seconds as you bend from your waist.
+ Pause for ½ second.
+ Exhale for 3 seconds as you slowly return to the starting position (maintaining a straight upper body).

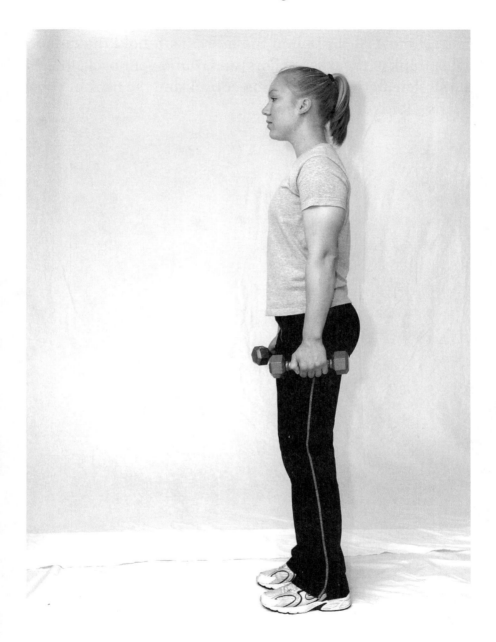

Figure 60. Dumbbell Deadlift (A)

Extra stretch: At the end of the movement, hold the dumb-bells (think of them as anchors) and round your back, to feel the stretch all through your lower back and the back of your thighs. Hold for 15 seconds.

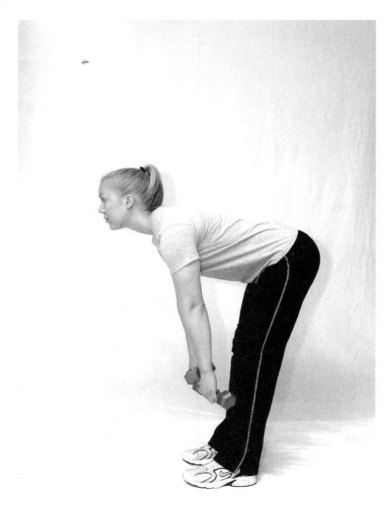

Figure 61. Dumbbell Deadlift (B)

Hints

✦ Start off using no weight.

✦ Make sure your movements are very slow and controlled.

✦ Feel a slight stretch in your hamstrings, but do not over stretch.

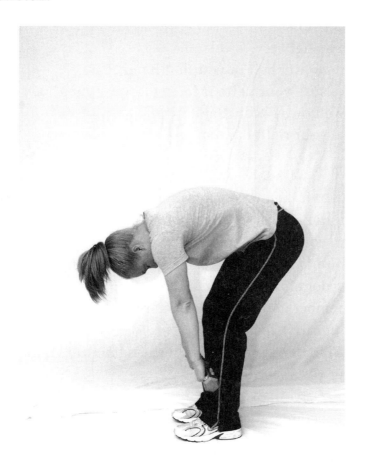

Figure 62. Dumbbell Stretch

for the middle of your shoulders

Dumbbell Side Raise

Position

+ Stand with your feet hip-width apart and your knees slightly bent.
+ Keep your shoulders back, chest out, and back straight with a slight forward lean.
+ Hold a dumbbell in your left hand.
+ Make sure your palm is facing toward your body, with your elbow slightly bent.
+ Place your right hand on your hip for balance.

Movement

+ Exhale, taking 3 seconds to raise the dumbbell away from the side of your body until it is at your shoulder level, your palms facing the floor.
+ Be sure to keep your wrist and elbow in line with your shoulder at the top of the movement.
+ Remember to think of pleasant thoughts as you let go of any negative feelings.
+ Pause for 2 seconds and feel the tightening in the middle of your shoulders.
+ Inhale as you lower the dumbbell in toward your body for 4 seconds.
+ Come down about three-quarters of the way.
+ Be sure not to let the dumbbell touch your body, as you will lose the tension.

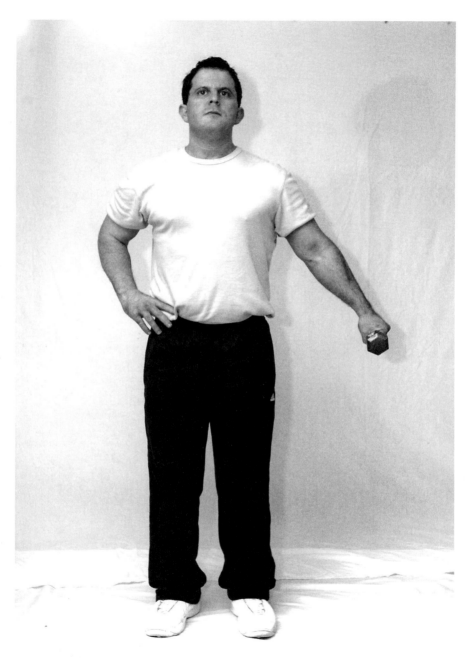

Figure 63. Dumbbell Side Raise (A)

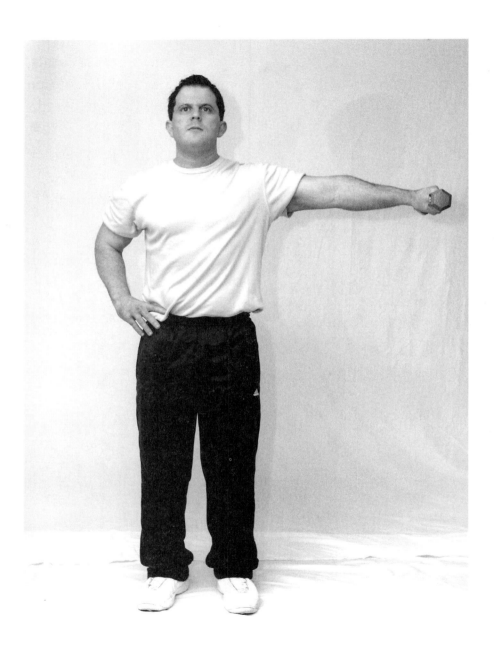

Figure 64. Dumbbell Side Raise (B)

Extra stretch: In order to get an extra stretch, hold the dumb-bell at the bottom and round your shoulders for 15 seconds, thinking of the weight as an anchor. As you feel the stretch in your shoulders, let your elbows shift slightly backward.

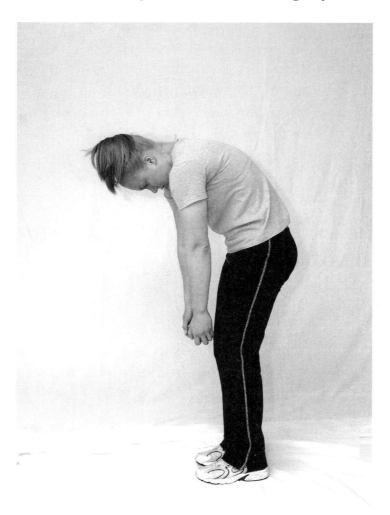

Figure 65. Rounded Shoulder Stretch

for the tops of your shoulders

Dumbbell Shoulder Shrugs

Position

+ Stand with your feet hip-width apart and your knees slightly bent.
+ Hold two dumbbells with arms extended down against your sides, palms facing your thighs.
+ Keep your shoulders back, chest out, and back straight with a forward lean.

Movement

+ Exhale, taking 3 seconds as you raise your shoulders as high as possible towards your ears.
+ Hold for 2 seconds at the top, feeling the top of your shoulders tightening.
+ Inhale for 4 seconds as you slowly lower the dumbbells to the starting position.

Extra stretch: At the end of the exercise, hold the dumbbells at your side and round your shoulders, feeling the top of your shoulders stretching.

Hold for 15 seconds.

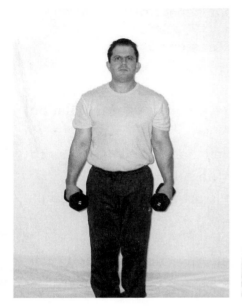 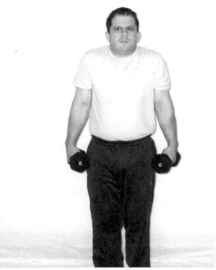

Figure 66. Dumbbell Shoulder Shrugs (A)   *Figure 67. Dumbbell Shoulder Shrugs (B)*

for the back of your upper arms

One-Arm Extensions

Position

- ✦ Sit on a chair with your back straight, your feet flat on the floor.
- ✦ Hold a dumbbell in your left hand by your ear with your elbow pointing out to the side.
- ✦ Keep your upper arm fixed (from shoulder to elbow).

Movement

- ✦ Exhale for 3 seconds as you raise the dumbbell (just moving your forearm) all the way up so your arm is straight.
- ✦ Hold for 2 seconds at the top, feeling the back of your upper arms tightening.
- ✦ Inhale for 4 seconds as you bring the dumbbell down.
- ✦ Bring the dumbbell down so that your arm forms an L shape, and your forearm is perpendicular to the floor.

Extra stretch: Stand straight with your knees slightly bent, feet shoulder-width apart, toes pointed straight ahead, shoulders level. Bend your left arm at your elbow with your upper arm next to your head and elbow pointing out.

Place your left fingers on top of your shoulders or back of your neck, then put your right hand on your left wrist. Pull gently to get an added stretch. Hold for 15 seconds. Repeat with your right arm.

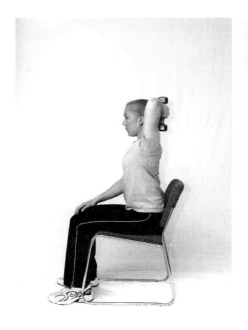

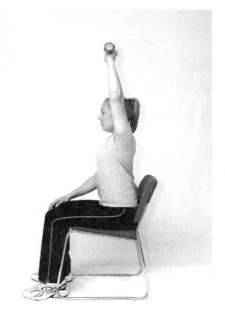

Figure 68. One-Arm Extensions (A)   *Figure 69. One-Arm Extensions (B)*

for the side of your upper arms

Kickbacks

Position

- Start with a light dumbbell in your left hand.
- Place your left foot on the ground.
- Bend at the waist and rest your right hand, arm straight, on a chair for support.
- Your back should be straight and parallel to the floor.
- Hold the dumbbell with your palm toward your body.
- Position your upper arm (from shoulder to elbow) so that it is parallel to the floor, elbow pointing back.
- Don't move your upper arm and keep the elbow close to your body.

Movement

- Exhale, taking 3 seconds as you extend the dumbbell back until your arm is straight and fully extended.
- Hold for 2 seconds, and feel the side of your upper arm tightening.
- Inhale for 4 seconds as you lower the weight.
- Bring the dumbbell down so that your arm forms an L shape, and your forearm is perpendicular to the floor.

Extra stretch: Bring the weight in toward your shoulder while keeping your elbow at your side, and feel the extra stretch in the back of your arm. Hold for 15 seconds. Repeat with your right arm.

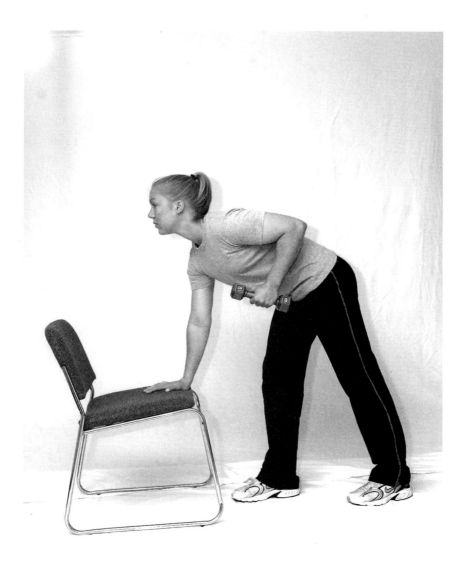

Figure 70. Kickbacks (A)

Caution

+ Don't bring the weight back too fast, or hyperextend your elbows. This will put too much strain on your elbow joint.

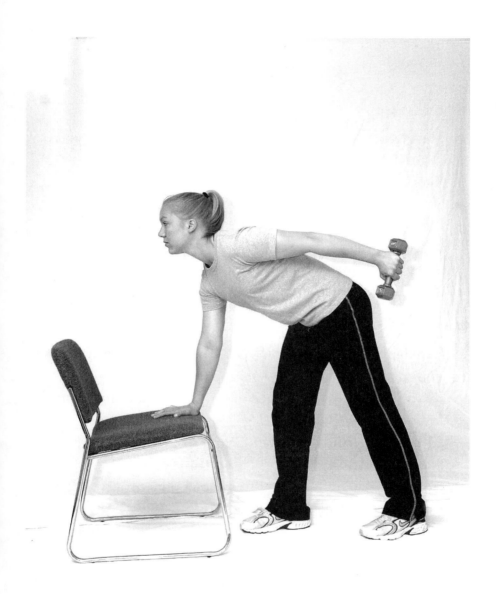

Figure 71. Kickbacks (A)

for the front of your upper arms (your biceps)

One-Arm Dumbbell Curls

Position

+ Stand with your feet hip-width apart and your knees slightly bent.
+ Keep your back straight and your stomach tight.
+ Start with a dumbbell in your left hand.
+ Place your right hand on your hip for balance.
+ Use an underhand grip.
+ Keep your upper arm (from elbow to shoulder) at your side throughout the movement and your wrist firm.

Movement

+ Exhale for 3 seconds as you curl the weight up towards your chest.
+ Keep your elbow fixed at your side, just moving your forearm.
+ At the top of the movement, your knuckles should be facing the ceiling.
+ Hold for 2 seconds at the top as you concentrate on the front of your upper arm tightening.
+ Inhale for 4 seconds as you slowly lower the dumbbell to the starting position.
+ Make sure you lower the dumbbell all the way down, but do not hyperextend your elbows.

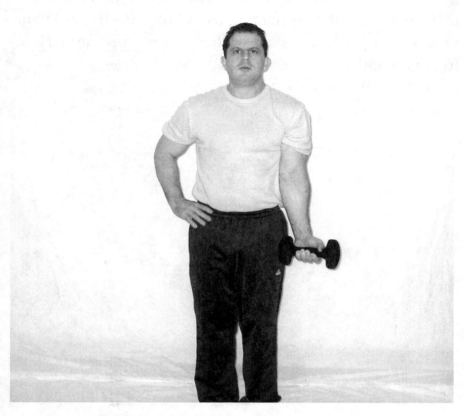

Figure 72. One-Arm Dumbbell Curls (A)

Extra stretch: At the end of the exercise, hold the dumbbell at the bottom of the movement, pause, then gently turn your wrist back to feel a fantastic stretch in your upper arm. Hold for 15 seconds.

Repeat with your right arm.

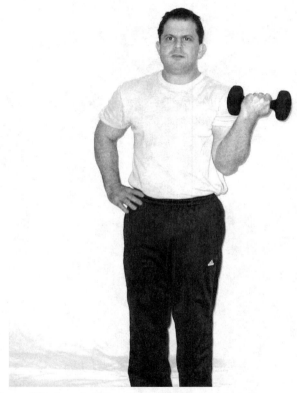

Figure 73. One-Arm Dumbbell Curls (B)

for the front of your upper arms

Concentration Curls

Position

+ With a dumbbell in your left hand, sit on an exercise bench or chair, with your feet about shoulder-width apart.
+ Bend forward and extend your left arm between your legs with your palm facing away from your body.
+ Keep your elbow and upper arm braced against the inside of your thigh.
+ Place your right hand onto your left upper arm just above the elbow for support.
+ Keep your upper arm fixed throughout the movement and your wrists firm.

Movement

+ Exhale, taking 3 seconds to curl the dumbbell up toward your shoulder.
+ Hold for 2 seconds at the top, feeling the front of your upper arm tightening.
+ Inhale for 4 seconds and slowly lower the weight to the starting position.
+ Make sure you lower the dumbbell all the way down, but do not hyperextend your elbows.

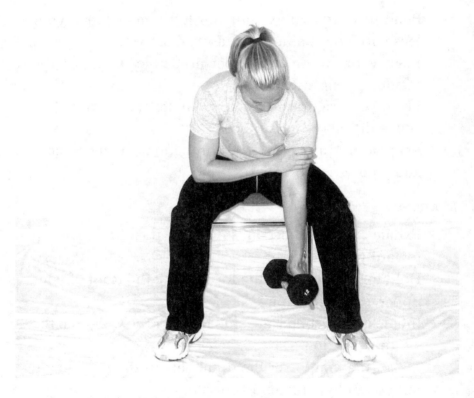

Figure 74. Concentration Curls (A)

Extra stretch: Turn your palm forward and your wrist back slightly to get an extra stretch. Hold for 15 seconds. Repeat with your right arm.

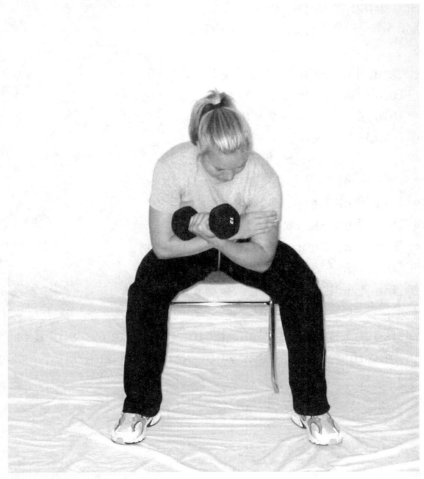

Figure 75. Concentration Curls (B)

Four-Week Advanced Program

Week 1

Schedule: 3 days per week,
Monday, Wednesday and Friday

+ Crunches with Feet Raised 2 x 8–15
+ Dumbbell Side Bend 1 x 8–12
+ Dumbbell Squats 2 x 8–12
+ Dumbbell Calf Raise 2 x 8–12
+ Dumbbell Bench Press 2 x 8–12
+ One-Arm Dumbbell Row 2 x 8–12
+ Dumbbell Deadlift 1 x 8–12
+ Dumbbell Side Raise 2 x 8–12
+ Dumbbell Shoulder Shrugs 1 x 8–12
+ One-Arm Extensions 2 x 8–12
+ One-Arm Dumbbell Curls 2 x 8–12

Walk for 2 minutes, then jog for 1 minute for a total of
20 minutes on Tuesday, Thursday, and Saturday.

Week 2

Schedule: 3 days per week,
Monday, Wednesday and Friday

* Crunches with Feet Raised 2 x 8–15
* Dumbbell Side Bend 1 x 8–12
* Dumbbell Squats 2 x 8–12
* Leg Extension with Ankle Weight 1 x 8–12
* Dumbbell Calf Raise 2 x 8–12
* Dumbbell Bench Press 2 x 8–12
* Incline Dumbbell Bench Press 1 x 8–12
* One-Arm Dumbbell Row 2 x 8–12
* Dumbbell Deadlift 2 x 8–12
* Dumbbell Side Raise 2 x 8–12
* Dumbbell Shoulder Shrugs 2 x 8–12
* One-Arm Extensions 2 x 8–12
* One-Arm Dumbbell Curls 2 x 8–12

Walk for 2 minutes, then jog for 2 minutes for a total of 20 minutes on Tuesday, Thursday, and Saturday.

Week 3

Schedule: 3 days per week,
Monday, Wednesday and Friday

+ Crunches with Feet Raised 2 x 8–15
+ Dumbbell Side Bend 2 x 8–12
+ Dumbbell Squats 2 x 8–12
+ Leg Extension with Ankle Weights 2 x 8–12
+ Leg Curl with Ankle Weights 1 x 8–12
+ Dumbbell Calf Raise 2 x 8–12
+ Dumbbell Bench Press 2 x 8–12
+ Incline Dumbbell Bench Press 2 x 8–12
+ One-Arm Dumbbell Row 2 x 8–12
+ Dumbbell Deadlift 2 x 8–12
+ Dumbbell Side Raise 2 x 8–12
+ Dumbbell Shoulder Shrugs 2 x 8–12
+ One-Arm Extensions 2 x 8–12
+ Kickbacks 1 x 8–12
+ One-Arm Dumbbell Curls 2 x 8–12
+ Concentration Curls 1 x 8–12

Walk for 1 minutes, then jog for 2 minutes for a total of 20
minutes on Tuesday, Thursday, and Saturday.

Week 4

Schedule: 3 days per week,
Monday, Wednesday and Friday

- Crunches with Feet Raised 2 x 8–15
- Dumbbell Side Bend 2 x 8–12
- Dumbbell Squats 2 x 8–12
- Leg Extension with Ankle Weights 2 x 8–12
- Leg Curl with Ankle Weights 2 x 8–12
- Dumbbell Calf Raise 2 x 8–12
- Dumbbell Bench Press 2 x 8–12
- Incline Dumbbell Bench Press 2 x 8–12
- One-Arm Dumbbell Row 2 x 8–12
- Dumbbell Deadlift 2 x 8–12
- Dumbbell Side Raise 2 x 8–12
- Dumbbell Shoulder Shrugs 2 x 8–12
- One-Arm Extensions 2 x 8–12
- Kickbacks 2 x 8–12
- One-Arm Dumbbell Curls 2 x 8–12
- Concentration Curls 2 x 8–12

Jog continuously for 20 minutes each day on Tuesday, Thursday, and Saturday.

Appendix I: Exercise List

Exercise Logs

Now that you've read about the Mindful Movements in this book, and it's likely you've already begun, my hope is you will commit to a program for at least four weeks. One of the best ways to keep you motivated is to track your progress.

The following worksheets will help you log your progress. You will be surprised by how wonderful even the lightest of workouts will make you feel, and there will be times that looking back at your progress will help you look forward.

You're on your way to a mind and body connection that will help you feel bet ter in so many aspects of your life. Congratulations for starting.

Strength-Training Log

Beginner Program—Week 1

Date _____ Time _____

In the white spaces below, fill in the number of repetitions you perform.

Exercise	Set # 1
Crunches	
Chair Squats	
Wall Push-Up	
Band Tricep Push-Down	
Band Bicep Curls	

Mood before: _____

Mood after: _____

Comments:

Weekly Aerobic Exercise Log

Beginner Program—Week 1

Day/Date	Type of Aerobic exercise	Planned Duration	Actual Duration	Mood Before	Mood After
	walk	5 minutes			
	walk	5 minutes			
	walk	5 minutes			

Strength-Training Log

Beginner Program—Week 2

Date _____   Time _____

In the white spaces below, fill in the number of repetitions you perform.

Exercise	Set # 1	Set # 2
Crunches		
Chair Squats		
Wall Push-Up		
Back Extension		
Band Tricep Push-Down		
Band Bicep Curls		

Mood before: _____

Mood after: _____

Comments:

Weekly Aerobic Exercise Log

Beginner Program—Week 2

Day/Date	Type of Aerobic exercise	Planned Duration	Actual Duration	Mood Before	Mood After
	walk	8 minutes			
	walk	8 minutes			
	walk	8 minutes			

Strength-Training Log

Beginner Program—Week 3

Date _____   Time _____

In the white spaces below, fill in the number of repetitions you perform.

Exercise	Set # 1	Set # 2
Crunches		
Chair Squats		
Wall Push-Up		
Back Extension		
Band Front Raise		
Band Tricep Push-Down		
Band Bicep Curls		

Mood before: _____

Mood after: _____

Comments:

Weekly Aerobic Exercise Log

Beginner Program—Week 3

Day/Date	Type of Aerobic exercise	Planned Duration	Actual Duration	Mood Before	Mood After
	walk	10 minutes			
	walk	10 minutes			
	walk	10 minutes			

Strength-Training Log

Beginner Program—Week 4

Date _____   Time _____

In the white spaces below, fill in the number of repetitions you perform.

Exercise	Set # 1	Set # 2
Crunches		
Chair Squats		
Wall Push-Up		
Back Extension		
Band Front Raise		
Band Tricep Push-Down		
Band Bicep Curls		

Mood before: _____

Mood after: _____

Comments:

Weekly Aerobic Exercise Log

Beginner Program—Week 4

Day/Date	Type of Aerobic exercise	Planned Duration	Actual Duration	Mood Before	Mood After
	walk	12 minutes			
	walk	12 minutes			
	walk	12 minutes			

Strength-Training Log

Intermediate Program—Week 1

Date _____ Time _____

In the white spaces below, fill in the number of repetitions you perform.

Exercise	Set # 1
Crunches with Feet Raised	
Body Weight Squats	
Standing Calf Raise	
Bent Knee Push-Up	
Band Seated Row	
Band Side Raise	
Band Reverse-Grip Tricep Push-Down	
Band Hammer Curls	

Mood before: _____

Mood after: _____

Comments:

Weekly Aerobic Exercise Log

Intermediate Program—Week 1

Day/Date	Type of Aerobic exercise	Planned Duration	Actual Duration	Mood Before	Mood After
	walk	15 minutes			
	walk	15 minutes			
	walk	15 minutes			

Strength-Training Log

Intermediate Program—Week 2

Date _____ Time _____

In the white spaces below, fill in the number of repetitions you perform.

Exercise	Set # 1	Set # 2
Crunches with Feet Raised		
Body Weight Squats		
Standing Calf Raise		
Bent Knee Push-Up		
Chest Crossover		
Band Seated Row		
Band Side Raise		
Band Reverse-Grip Tricep Push-Down		
Band Hammer Curls		

Mood before: _____

Mood after: _____

Comments:

Weekly Aerobic Exercise Log

Intermediate Program—Week 2

Day/Date	Type of Aerobic exercise	Planned Duration	Actual Duration	Mood Before	Mood After
	walk	18 minutes			
	walk	18 minutes			
	walk	18 minutes			

Strength-Training Log

Intermediate Program—Week 3

Date _____   Time _____

In the white spaces below, fill in the number of repetitions you perform.

Exercise	Set # 1	Set # 2
Crunches with Feet Raised		
Body Weight Squats		
Single Leg Standing Calf Raise		
Standard Push-Up		
Chest Crossover		
Band Seated Row		
Band Side Raise		
Band Reverse-Grip Tricep Push-Down		
Band Hammer Curls		

Mood before: _____

Mood after: _____

Comments:

Weekly Aerobic Exercise Log

Intermediate Program—Week 3

Day/Date	Type of Aerobic exercise	Planned Duration	Actual Duration	Mood Before	Mood After
	walk	20 minutes			
	walk	20 minutes			
	walk	20 minutes			

Strength-Training Log

Intermediate Program—Week 4

Date _____   Time _____

In the white spaces below, fill in the number of repetitions you perform.

Exercise	Set # 1	Set # 2
Crunches with Feet Raised		
Body Weight Squats		
Single Leg Standing Calf Raise		
Standard Push-Up		
Chest Crossover		
Band Seated Row		
Band Side Raise		
Band Reverse-Grip Tricep Push-Down		
Band Hammer Curls		

Mood before: _____

Mood after: _____

Comments:

Weekly Aerobic Exercise Log

Intermediate Program—Week 4

Day/Date	Type of Aerobic exercise	Planned Duration	Actual Duration	Mood Before	Mood After
	alternate walking for 2 minutes with jogging for 30 seconds	20 minutes			
	alternate walking for 2 minutes with jogging for 30 seconds	20 minutes			
	alternate walking for 2 minutes with jogging for 30 seconds	20 minutes			

Strength-Training Log

Advanced Program—Week 1

Date _____   Time _____

In the white spaces below, fill in the weight and number of repetitions you perform. For example, 5 x 9 equals 5 lbs. for 9 repetitions.

Exercise	Set # 1	Set # 2
Crunches with Feet Raised		
Dumbbell Side Bends		
Dumbbell Squats		
Dumbbell Calf Raise		
Dumbbell Bench Press		
One-Arm Row		
Dumbbell Deadlift		
Dumbbell Side Raise		
Dumbbell Shoulder Shrugs		
One-Arm Extensions		
One-Arm Dumbbell Curls		

Mood before: _____

Mood after: _____

Comments:

Weekly Aerobic Exercise Log

Advanced Program—Week 1

Day/Date	Type of Aerobic exercise	Planned Duration	Actual Duration	Mood Before	Mood After
	alternate walking for 2 minutes with jogging for 1 minute	20 minutes			
	aAlternate walking for 2 minutes with jogging for 1 minute	20 minutes			
	alternate walking for 2 minutes with jogging for 1 minute	20 minutes			

Strength-Training Log

Advanced Program—Week 2

Date _____   Time _____

In the white spaces below, fill in the weight and number of repetitions you perform. For example, 5 x 9 equals 5 lbs. for 9 repetitions.

Exercise	Set # 1	Set # 2
Crunches with Feet Raised		
Dumbbell Side Bend		
Dumbbell Squats		
Leg Extensions with Ankle Weights		
Dumbbell Calf Raise		
Dumbbell Bench Press		
Incline Dumbbell Bench Press		
One-Arm Dumbbell Row		
Dumbbell Deadlift		
Dumbbell Side Raise		
Dumbbell Shoulder Shrugs		
One-Arm Extensions		
One-Arm Dumbbell Curls		

Mood before: _____

Mood after: _____

Comments:

Weekly Aerobic Exercise Log

Advanced Program—Week 2

Day/Date	Type of Aerobic exercise	Planned Duration	Actual Duration	Mood Before	Mood After
	alternate walking for 2 minutes with jogging for 2 minutes	20 minutes			
	alternate walking for 2 minutes with jogging for 2 minutes	20 minutes			
	alternate walking for 2 minutes with jogging for 2 minutes	20 minutes			

Strength-Training Log

Advanced Program—Week 3

Date _____ Time _____

In the white spaces below, fill in the weight and number of repetitions you perform. For example, 5 x 9 equals 5 lbs. for 9 repetitions.

Exercise	Set # 1	Set # 2
Crunches with Feet Raised		
Dumbbell Side Bend		
Dumbbell Squats		
Leg Extensions with Ankle Weights		
Leg Curls with Ankle Weights		
Dumbbell Calf Raise		
Dumbbell Bench Press		
Incline Dumbbell Bench Press		
One-Arm Dumbbell Row		
Dumbbell Deadlift		
Dumbbell Side Raise		
Dumbbell Shoulder Shrugs		
One-Arm Extensions		
Kickbacks		
One-Arm Dumbbell Curls		
Concentration Curls		

Mood before: _____

Mood after: _____

Comments:

Weekly Aerobic Exercise Log

Advanced Program—Week 3

Day/Date	Type of Aerobic exercise	Planned Duration	Actual Duration	Mood Before	Mood After
	alternate walking for 1 minutes with jogging for 2 minutes	20 minutes			
	alternate walking for 1 minutes with jogging for 2 minutes	20 minutes			
	alternate walking for 1 minutes with jogging for 2 minutes	20 minutes			

Strength-Training Log

Advanced Program—Week 4

Date _____   Time _____

In the white spaces below, fill in the weight and number of repetitions you perform. For example, 5 x 9 equals 5 lbs. for 9 repetitions.

Exercise	Set # 1	Set # 2
Crunches with Feet Raised		
Dumbbell Side Bend		
Dumbbell Squats		
Leg Extensions with Ankle Weights		
Leg Curls with Ankle Weights		
Dumbbell Calf Raise		
Dumbbell Bench Press		
Incline Dumbbell Bench Press		
One-Arm Dumbbell Row		
Dumbbell Deadlift		
Dumbbell Side Raise		
Dumbbell Shoulder Shrugs		
One-Arm Extensions		
Kickbacks		
One-Arm Dumbbell Curls		
Concentration Curls		

Mood before: _____

Mood after: _____

Comments:

Weekly Aerobic Exercise Log

Advanced Program—Week 4

Day/Date	Type of Aerobic exercise	Planned Duration	Actual Duration	Mood Before	Mood After
	Jog	20 minutes			
	Jog	20 minutes			
	Jog	20 minutes			

Resources

Self-Help Books

Bernie Siegel, M.D., *Love, Medicine & Miracles*, HarperCollins Publishers, 1988

Bernie Siegel, M.D., *365 Prescriptions for the Soul*, New World Library, 2003

David Burns, M.D., *Feeling Good Handbook*, Plume Publishing, 1999

Harrison G. Pope, M.D., Katherine A. Phillips, M.D., Roberto Olivardia, M.D., *The Adonis Complex*, Simon & Schuster Adult Publishing Group, 2002

Lisa Berger, Alexander Vuckovic, M.D., *Under Observation*, Penguin Publishing, 1995

Fitness Books

Wayne Westcott, Ph.D., *Strength Training Past 50*, Human Kinetics Publishers, 1997

JoAnn Manson, M.D., Patricia Amend, *30-Minute Fitness Solution: A Four-Step Plan for Women of All Ages,* Harvard University Press, 2001

Nutrition Books

Walter C. Willett, M.D., *Eat, Drink, and Be Healthy: The Harvard Medical School Guide to Healthy Eating*, Simon & Schuster Adult Publishing Group, 2002
Andrew Stoll, M.D., *The Omega-3 Connection,* Simon & Schuster Adult Publishing Group, 2002

Equipment

SPRI Products
800-222-7774
www.spriproducts.com

PowerBlocks®
800-446-5215
www.powerblock.com

PlateMates®
800-877-3322
www.theplatemate.com

Index

emotional healing
   Sarah's achievement of 47 – 48
endorphins 13, 35
energy improvement and stress
  relief
   Susan's achievement of 46 – 47
enkephalins 13, 35
equipment
   ankle weights, adjustable 149
   dumbbells 149
   heavy pole 84
   step, adjustable 149
   weight bench 149
Evans, Richard L. 75
exercise
   rubber exercise bands 92
exercise bands, rubber 92
extensions
   back 102
   leg with ankle weights 156
   one-arm 186

fats 59 – 60
Fitchburg State College 21
four-week programs
   advanced 198 – 201
   beginning 110 – 113
   intermediate 145 – 148
Fran's success 49 – 50
functional fitness 66 – 67

George's success 44 – 45
Gleason, Amy 54 – 62
gradual progressions 70 – 73
guilt about not exercising 40
gyms, local
   no pain, no gain philosophy 28
   problems with 26, 38

habit
   establishing exercise 39 – 41, 62
herbs 61

intermediate four-week program
  145 – 148
isolated movement 69

jogging 74
junk food and mood 53 – 54

Keller, Helen 43
Kennedy, John F. 149
kickbacks 188

legs
   dumbbell deadlift 176
   standing calf stretch 80
Lincoln, Abraham 19
listening to your muscles 65

macho weightlifters 45
marijuana 21
meal size and frequency 57 – 59
mental relapse prevention 36
mindful movements 16 – 17, 63 – 66
moderation 70, 73
mood
   and Aspartame 58
   and caffeine 53 – 56
   and diet 53 – 54
   and exercise 35
mood (continued)
   and meal size and frequency 57 – 59
   and protein 57
   and steroids 22

and strength training 26, 27
and sugar 53 – 54
movement definitions 68 – 69
muscle group order 71

negative movement 69
no pain, no gain philosophy 19,
    28, 51, 64

one-arm dumbell curls 192
one-arm extension 186

peak contraction 68
physical strength and balance
    George's achievement of 44 – 46
positive movement 68
positive reinforcement 41
protein 56 – 57
push-downs
    band tricep 106
    reverse-grip tricep 140
push-ups
    bent-knee 126
    standard 128
    wall 98

raises
    band front 104
    band side 136
    dumbbell calf 164
    dumbbell side 180
    single-leg 124
    single-leg calf 124
    standing calf 122
Randolph, Massachusetts 20
repetition 68
reps 68

reverse-grip tricep push-down 140
'roid rages 22
Rousseau, Jean Jacques 91
rows
    band seated 134
    one-arm dumbbell 172
rubber exercise bands 92

Sarah's success 47 – 48
serotonin 57
set 68
shoulder shrugs
    dumbbell 184
shoulders
    band front raise 104
    band side raise 136
    chest and shoulder stretch 82,
        126, 128
    dumbbell shoulder shrugs 184
    dumbbell side raise 180
sleep
    and caffeine 55
    and exercise 13, 62
snack
    before exercising 40, 61
squats
    bodyweight 118
    chair 95
    dumbbell 154
standing calf stretch 80
standing hamstring stretch 78
standing quadricep stretch 77
step, adjustable 149
steroids 21, 31
    addiction to 19 – 23
    and aggressive behavoir 22
    easy availability of 22
    'roid rages 22

About the Author

For over 15 years, Jeff Rutstein, president of Custom Fitness, has been providing personal strength training for a diverse population coping with a broad range of challenges:

+ Patients referred by their mental health counselor as part of a clinical treatment program
+ High profile professionals seeking to manage their everyday stress for greater productivity
+ Adults, young and old, who are recovering from alcohol and drug abuse.

Jeff was named Distinguished Personal Trainer by *American Fitness,* an Outstanding Fitness Leader by *Reebok Instructor News,* The Best Samaritan by *American Health,* and is a Master Level Personal Trainer certified by the International Dance and Exercise Association (IDEA). Jeff has shared his experiences and fitness program on ABC and

NBC, in *The Washington Post,* Reuters, *The Boston Globe, Natural Health,* and dozens of other media outlets.

Jeff took courses in psychology, exercise science, and nutrition in college—useful in his job as a fitness specialist, but most of what he needed to know came from his life experiences. Jeff started drinking at age 12, and by age 22, was physically addicted to alcohol, several street drugs, and steroids. Trying to quit cold turkey, he was hospitalized when his pulse rate hit 144 at rest—heart attack level.

When Jeff stopped using drugs and alcohol, he found himself in a powerful depression; he was in a black hole that felt inescapable. Going back to his passion for weightlifting, but without steroids or other drugs, strength training played an essential role in his recovery and also led to his discovery of the techniques he describes in *Rutstein on Fitness,* Jeff's recovery, replacing depression with self-esteem and a new sense of physical and mental fitness, motivated him to share his method with others.

In 1990, he started a personal training center based on a complete mind-body approach to exercise that can be meditative while reducing stress, increasing self-esteem and total fitness. His efforts blossomed after a number of leading physicians and mental health professionals heard about his work and began to refer patients to him. *Rutstein on Fitness* is the result of a lifetime of experience and Jeff's deep desire to help the millions of others throughout the world who are dealing with everyday stress or the more daunting prospect of recovering from depression and addiction.